Cardio Kickboxing® Elite

Cardio Kickboxing® Elite

For Sport
For Fitness
For Self-Defense

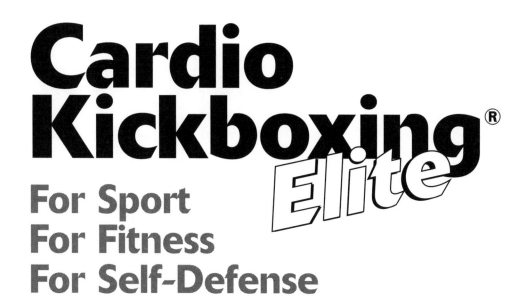

Frank Thiboutot

YMAA PUBLICATION CENTER
Boston, Mass. USA

YMAA Publication Center
Main Office:
4354 Washington Street
Boston, Massachusetts, 02131
617-323-7215 • ymaa@aol.com • www.ymaa.com

10 9 8 7 6 5 4 3 2 1

ISBN:1-886969-92-2

Edited by Sharon Rose
Cover design by Richard Rossiter

Publisher's Cataloging in Publication

(Prepared by Quality Books Inc.)

Thiboutot, Frank.
　　Cardio kickboxing elite : for sport, for fitness, for
self-defense / by Frank Thiboutot -- 1st ed.
　　p. cm.
　　Includes bibliographical references and index.
　　LCCN: 00-106041
　　ISBN: 1-886969-92-2

　　1. Physical fitness.　2. Kickboxing.　I. Title.

RA781.T45 2001　　　　　　613.7'148
　　　　　　　　　　　　　　　QBI00-791

Disclaimer:
The author and publisher of this material are NOT RESPONSIBLE in any manner whatsoever for any injury which may occur through reading or following the instructions in this manual.
The activities, physical or otherwise, described in this material may be too strenuous or dangerous for some people, and the reader(s) should consult a physician before engaging in them.

Printed in Canada.

Dedication

This book is dedicated to all amateur and professional kickboxers as well as the trainers, managers, promoters, and officials who have been involved in the development of the sport of kickboxing especially in North America. These fighters may not be household names as far as the general public is concerned, but they had an impact on the transition from traditional martial arts to Full Contact Karate, which is now known as "kickboxing". In the mid-seventies and early eighties there was Joe Lewis, Jeff Smith, Bill Wallace, Brad Hefton, Benny Urquidez, Anthony Elmore, Paul Vizzio, Jerry Trimble, and Howard Jackson. In the eighties and nineties Bob Thurman, Maurice Smith, Jean-Ives Theriault, Dennis Alexio, Curtis Bush, Don Wilson, Rick Roufus, Pete Cunningham, Mike Miles, Jose Torres, my personal favorite Danny Melendez, and countless others helped continue the mission.

Look for fighters like Alex Gong, Jean-Claude Leuyer, Olando Rivera, and Cung Lee to lead the sport in the new millennium (the real millennium in 2001). The sport has made great strides overseas especially in The Netherlands, (Rob Kaman) the UK, (Trevor Ambrose), the former Soviet Union, (Alexei Nechaev and Vitaly Klitchko) and Australia (Stan Longinidis) where the game has been greatly influenced by Muay Thai. As it should be, the world ratings of the leading sanctioning bodies are now filled with fighters from all over the world rather than just North America.

Furthermore, some fighters have actually won titles in both boxing and kickboxing. Kaosai Galaxy and Samart Payakaroon won Muay Thai titles in Thailand and then world titles in boxing. Nigel Benn of England was a Thai boxing champion in the U.K. before becoming a world champion in boxing. In the U.S., Troy Dorsey and James Warring won world American-style kickboxing titles first and then won world boxing titles later on in their careers.

Hopefully, as *Cardio Kickboxing*® increases in popularity as an awesome fitness program, it will continue to bring more attention to the sport.

Table of Contents

Foreword

The fitness industry is in the midst of tackling the Surgeon General's challenge to increase the physical activity of Americans. As such, it is evolving to become more inclusive of a wide variety of populations. Greater emphasis is being placed on programs that are based on scientifically sound exercise principles. In our culture's belated pursuit of the mind-body connection, the industry is attempting to address the "whole" person with mind-body programming. In a continuing effort to help participants find activities they find enjoyable, a wide variety of programming has been undertaken.

Cardio Kickboxing® Elite is suitable for all ages and abilities, males and females alike, those who want to compete and those who have general health and fitness goals in mind.

With the aging of our population, it is important to provide opportunities for older individuals to begin or continue to stay active. Many of us "boomers" have grown up in a culture of active living and are looking for additional ways to continue that lifestyle, and to do it in a social setting. Martial arts programs have been promoted as a way to enhance physical skills and fitness and to promote confidence of youth. Furthering that effort, this program is based on sound fitness development principles and provides for progressive mastery of skills. In the 1980s and for much of the 1990s, group exercise had pretty much been the exclusive domain of females. With the need for variety and the desire to offer programs attractive to males, exercise programming has become diversified to include such classes as "Boot Camp," sports conditioning classes, and martial arts sans equipment based exercise classes. Here in the year 2000, these programs have continued to attract greater numbers of females relative to males. With the equipment emphasis of this program, the appeal may increase for males.

Frank Thiboutot has developed a program that effectively partners the medium of kickboxing with sound exercise principles, a critical union that has been overlooked by many of the exercise videos and products available in the market today.

He has been prudent in addressing the American College of Sports Medicine's (ACSM) guidelines for developing and maintaining cardiorespiratory and muscular fitness. By participating in this program, individuals can improve their aerobic fitness levels, enhance muscular strength and endurance, increase flexibility and improve body composition (less fat, more muscle). With lack of time being the most common barrier to exercise and physical activity, *Cardio Kickboxing® Elite* effectively addresses these components in one comprehensive session.

Cardio Kickboxing® Elite effectively addresses the "whole" person. This is a "hot" area in the fitness industry today as evidenced by the increase in popularity of yoga, Tai Chi, and Pilates, as well as the inclusion of relaxation techniques in mainstream exercise classes. While the physical aspect of this program is obvious, less so are the positive influences on the psychological, social, and spiritual dimensions of the individual. In addition to increasing knowledge of the kickboxing sport and general fitness principles, potential psychological benefits of participating in this program include reduction of stress, reduction of anxiety and depression, and enhancement of self-esteem. By following Frank's recommendations to undertake this program in a group setting, numerous social needs can be met. Lastly, if so moved, each individual can find a way to integrate this program with his or her own spiritual dimension.

While people may start to become more physically active for health benefits, the primary reason that people maintain active lifestyles is enjoyment, an element that is crucial to continued motivation and adherence. With a much wider variety of group exercise programming than was available a mere ten years ago, there is a much greater chance that individuals will find that one activity that meets their needs and that they enjoy. For those of us already living an active lifestyle, *Cardio Kickboxing® Elite* can serve as an adjunct to our ongoing exercise programs, offering that much needed cross-training. For beginning and experienced exercisers alike, this program can become the foundation for which other programs supplement. For those of you who already train or compete in the sport of kickboxing, training in a group setting can provide some additional motivation, camaraderie, and competitiveness.

Cardio Kickboxing® Elite is an exciting new program that will help individuals begin and continue to lead active, healthy lifestyles. Having been in the fitness industry for nearly 20 years and having participated in physical activity since prior to leaving the womb, I personally commit to expanding my "dabbling" in this medium to more active involvement.

Karen Croteau, Ed.D.
Assistant Professor of Sports Medicine
University of Southern Maine

Preface

I have had almost four decades of experience in the martial arts, twenty-three years of which involved the sport of American-style kickboxing, formerly known as full-contact karate. In 1992, I created the original *Cardio Kickboxing®* workout program. The primary objective was to promote the *sport* of kickboxing through kickboxing for *fitness*. My mission was and always has been to safely mainstream the workout of a fighter to the general public for its fitness and self-defense benefits. Thus, this program has always focused on *sport-specific* techniques used in boxing, kickboxing, and Thai-style boxing. It has also always been equipment intensive. Would you want to play basketball without a ball or a hoop? How much fun would that be? Using conventional boxing and kickboxing training tools, such as heavy bags, uppercut bags, double-end bags, punch mitts, focus pads, etc., provides:

1. a *resistance* component to an already demanding cardiovascular workout for greater fitness benefits, and;

2. techniques that are authentic and efficient so that they could be effective for self-defense purposes.

In order to introduce this workout concept to the market, I approached a number of fitness video companies to produce a video for me, but there was no interest at the time. Consequently, I self-produced the *Cardio Kickboxing®*, *"The Workout with a Kick!"* video in 1993 as well as registered 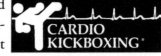 the name and trademark. I always believed this workout concept would be a hit. With a lot of hard work at the grassroots level sending out hundreds of press releases and complimentary preview copies of the video to various media sources, doing countless demos and interviews, I found that, eight years later, it became an *overnight* success.

Over time, the *Cardio Kickboxing®* workout as well as a number of other *fitness Kickboxing®* programs became an *alternative* to conventional aerobics, now called group fitness classes. Initially, the aerobics industry was not interested in working with my company to help develop a certification program so, as I did with my first video, we developed our own. We have certified hundreds of instructors here in the U.S. and overseas. Now that it has been demonstrated that the public is, in fact, interested in martial arts based workouts for fitness, the aerobics industry has seen the wisdom of developing and offering their own instructor certifications for "kickboxing". However, their approach to certifying instructors in "kickboxing" comes into question for two reasons: 1) instructors are certified in a weekend workshops and 2) eliminating the roundhouse kick because they believe it is "unsafe". Does it make sense to eliminate the most widely used kick in kickboxing especially in Thai boxing? Or, should they find a way to teach this kick properly to minimize the risk of injury?

The *Cardio Kickboxing®* program is grounded in techniques from the sport of kickboxing as well as martial arts. Having worked in the fitness industry myself, I certainly recognized the need for tailoring the program to meet the needs of those who were not necessarily as physically fit or as young as some of the competitive fighters I had worked with over the years. I also recognize that there are space and budget limitations in health clubs and martial arts schools, so we also began offering a "without" equipment option for our instructors. However, they are still required to go through and pass the "with" equipment components *first* and are then allowed to dovetail off of the original program. With so many people having already been exposed to boxing, kickboxing, and martial arts who might wind up in their classes, they had better know their stuff to maintain their credibility as instructors.

Unlike some traditional martial arts instructors who would never consider deviating from how they were taught by their teachers we actually encourage our prospective instructors to bring their own personalities and styles of presentation into the mix based on their backgrounds and teaching experiences. Otherwise, to do things my way only would certainly stifle creativity. Instead of just mimicking the moves, we provide them with the bio-mechanically correct knowledge of how to throw a punch or kick as well as an understanding of the terminology, jargon, and history of how the program evolved from a sport into a fitness program. Learning these basic and fundamental concepts has enabled our instructors to be better qualified and more confident when teaching.

Even though I felt this workout concept would be a success, I never envisioned it would become as big as it has. *Cardio Kickboxing®* has spawned many hybrid programs, some of which are more aerobics rather than kickboxing oriented. Many former aerobic instructors are even producing their own "kickboxing" videos. However, there has been a recent tendency by some *aerobic kickboxing* instructors to water-down the original program and simply make up movements so that they will fit neatly and tidily into an aerobics class format that conforms to the beat of the music. This is not necessary with all the additional intermediate and advanced techniques available from the sport of kickboxing.

Even though the origins of kickboxing can be traced back to ancient China, I have found that many traditional martial artists lack an in-depth knowledge of current conditioning and safety standards that is of utmost priority justifiably demanded by the health and fitness industry. Conversely, the health and fitness industry—which is really still in its infancy, by comparison, having come into its own only about three or four decades ago—knows little about kickboxing. My secondary goal of helping to bring these two industries together is beginning to be realized.

Acknowledgements

Thanks to my instructor Seung-Ook Choi who convinced me that in order to excel in the sport of kickboxing, you need to practice the sport-specific techniques that work in the ring. His favorite saying is, "Practice does not make perfect; *perfect* practice makes perfect."

And thanks to Rush Limbaugh who inspired me to produce my first video in 1993 and then develop the instructor certification program in 1996, even though I had no previous experience in either of these two areas.

A special thanks to my wife, Judie, who put up with my desire over the past eight years to help change the way the martial arts are taught in this country.

And lastly, a special thank you to my son, Garik, who aspires to become a golf pro—the inspiration for me to write this book. How else am I going to pay for his lessons?

> *If I believe I cannot do something, it makes me incapable of doing it. But when I believe I can, then I acquire the ability to do it, even if I did not have the ability in the beginning.*
>
> *—Mahatma Gandhi*

The kickboxing community extends its appreciation to all promoters, but especially to Bruce and Cindy Marshall. Over the years, they have had every imaginable roadblock thrown up in front of them as well as one financial setback after the other trying to promote the sport, but NEVER gave up. They possess the same nose to the grindstone, never say die, risk-taking characteristics of the countless people who made this country great. (That does not mean Hollywood celebrities, the MTV crowd, liberal politicians, the mainstream media or high profile, whiney, overpaid ball players). **They have the true warrior spirit.**

Purpose

The purpose of this book is to provide you with all you will need to know about *Cardio Kickboxing®*. Not only is *Cardio Kickboxing®* a great means for improving your health by increasing your fitness level, but as a by-product of the workout, you will be learning valuable self-defense techniques.

The book will give you a brief history of the origins of martial arts, how the martial arts evolved into the sport of kickboxing and how the sport was developed into a fitness program. You will be given detailed information on the fundamentals needed and a workout a kickboxer would use to improve his conditioning and skill level. This is followed by intermediate and advanced techniques that will further enhance your knowledge of kickboxing. There are subsequent optional workouts that you can use for increasing cardiovascular endurance. Also provided are recommendations on equipment, instructions describing how that equipment is used, and explanations of how the equipment develops skill, power, and the ability to effectively utilize the punches and kicks you have learned on actual targets. Finally, the book is an additional resource guide for music, videos, and certification programs that are available to take the program to whatever level you wish.

Although the book was designed for those who are just getting started, it will prove very beneficial if you are already participating in martial arts style group fitness classes and want a deeper understanding of the application of the techniques you are learning. It will also be a must read if you prefer to work out in the privacy and convenience of your own home.

Although there really is not much that is new in the sport of kickboxing, the training methodology does change, however. Spending 3–4 hours a day in a gym to actually train like a professional kickboxer is unrealistic for most adults who have regular jobs, families to raise and a multitude of other everyday priorities. The *Cardio Kickboxing®* workout, which has now been time tested in the marketplace for eight years, can be done in a 45–60 minute session. It is a safe and effective step-by-step exercise program developed to meet the needs of the general population.

No doubt, you have seen countless infomercials or ads in supermarket tabloids touting one workout or diet after another that guarantees results with little effort. I am here to tell you up front, it is *not* going to happen. However, you might find this program interesting enough to take the first step to better fitness.

Introduction

My longtime motto with regards to exercise is that, *it does not matter WHAT you do as long as you DO something*. However, to only do activities like jogging or riding a stationary bike would be too one-dimensional to suit me as well as a lot of other people. A single program that offers variety will help ensure that your motivational level stays high. Because *Cardio Kickboxing*® offers so many techniques to learn and the classes may change somewhat even on a daily basis, it is never boring. When you're on the equipment circuit, for example, you can also work at your own skill and fitness level. There's so much going on in a *Cardio Kickboxing*® class that you sometimes do not even realize you're getting a great workout until after class is over.

If you cannot find the time to get to a class or prefer to exercise in the comfort and privacy of your own home, you can also benefit from this workout. Initially, you can go through the warm-up routine and review the punches, kicks, and combinations. You can also do a number of shadow boxing and shadow kickboxing rounds and gradually increase the number of rounds you do on a given day. Learn how to skip rope and then do your cool-down and stretches to complete your workout.

The next step would be to purchase and install a heavy bag that you can hang in your garage or basement. If you live in an apartment, you could purchase a freestanding heavy bag instead. You could also invest in some skill-oriented bags such as a double-end bag that does not take up much space. By adding the resistance and skill bags to your routine, *you will* be well on your way to seeing increased fitness results as well as feeling better about yourself. Initially, I would recommend that you do your *Cardio Kickboxing*® workout two to three times per week and maybe add some jogging, ride a bike, or climb on a Stairmaster on your alternate days.

Since I have been doing this type of workout for so many years, I sometimes forget that it is second nature to me but suggest you do what I did when I took up golf. Get a good grasp of the fundamentals FIRST making sure what you learn is bio-mechanically sound and then go out and play. Practice, polish, and play and then do that sequence over again. It is the only way to master and become proficient at anything, especially kickboxing.

For what it is worth, I have never been on a supermarket tabloid diet and eat pretty much whatever I want. I have also never purchased an AB Roller or any other piece of exercise equipment from a TV infomercial. When I took a recent physical, my doctor said I had the blood pressure and resting heart rate of a teenager. My HDL (good) cholesterol was off the charts. When I took a cursory fitness test I took on the treadmill, I plugged in the age of 25, which indicated my level of cardiovascular conditioning was "excellent." In December 1999, I turned 50. Forget those bogus celebrity testimonials and let us get started with the program that will really make a difference in your health and fitness.

In Summary. Kenneth H. Cooper, M.D., M.P.H. is credited with coining the term "aerobics".

"In 1968 *Aerobics* was published in an effort to make the American people more aware of their need for exercise and to encourage them to use exercise in the practice of preventative medicine." Dr. Cooper's research was primarily conducted on young U.S. military personnel. Two years later, *The New Aerobics* was published emphasizing age adjusted endurance-type activities with an emphasis on safety. In 1970, Dr. Cooper founded The Institute for Aerobics Research where thousands of patients have since been evaluated and medically prescribed exercise programs.

In the seventies, the fledgling fitness industry had begun to supplant the traditional YMCA, YWCA, and Boys Clubs with health clubs for those seeking improved fitness and recreation in a group setting. Aerobic classes were given a boost in attention by Jane Fonda videos that came into vogue. Dance oriented in design, these classes appealed especially to women who recognized the value of regular exercise. Since the mid-eighties, organizations such as ACE (American Council on Exercise) and AFAA (Aerobics and Fitness Association of America) have certified thousands of instructors to safely and professionally conduct these types of classes for the general public who were both fit and unfit. In 1999, there were approximately 13,300 health clubs in the United States that have approximately 46,000,000 members.

According to *A Report of the Surgeon General, Physical Activity and Health, 1996*:

- People who are usually inactive can improve their health and wellbeing by becoming at least moderately active on a regular basis.
- Physical activity need not be strenuous to achieve health benefits.
- Greater health benefits can be achieved by increasing the amount (duration, frequency, or intensity) of physical activity.
- Regular physical activity performed on most days of the week improves health in the following ways:
- Reduces the risk of dying prematurely.
- Reduces the risk of dying from heart disease.
- Reduces the risk of developing diabetes.

- Reduces the risk of developing high blood pressure.
- Helps reduce blood pressure in people who already have high blood pressure.
- Reduces the risk of developing colon cancer.
- Reduces the feelings of depression and cancer.
- Reduces the feelings of depression and anxiety.
- Helps control weight.
- Helps build and maintain healthy bones, muscles, and joints.
- Helps older adults become stronger and better able to move about without falling.
- Promotes psychological wellbeing.

By now it should not be a secret that exercise is good for you. Yet, the same report states:

- More than 60 percent of adults do not achieve the recommended amount of regular physical activity. In fact, 25 percent of all adults are not active at all.
- Nearly half of young people aged 12 to 21 are not vigorously active on a regular basis.
- In high school, enrollment in daily physical education classes has dropped from 42 percent in 1991 to 25 percent in 1995.

It is clear from the above information that:

1. For those who are not exercising at all, that you have to take the first step to get started in some type of program. As I mentioned in the earlier, it does not matter what you do for exercise as long as you do something. There are no shortcuts as touted by the numerous infomercials *you will* see on television. Low to moderate intensity workouts can improve your health; however, for increased fitness benefits, you can gradually increase the frequency and intensity and duration of your workouts. It is a simple formula. Move more; eat less. It is your good health that's at stake.

2. For those who are already involved in an exercise regimen whether it be aerobics, jogging, Spinning®, and so on, you've recognized that there is value in incorporating fitness into your lifestyle not just as a New Year's resolution. But, are you working out at an appropriate level to increase your level of fitness or are you mainly socializing? And if you are, in fact, working out, how do you stay motivated?

You need a regimen that provides an efficient cardiovascular and resistance workout that is interesting, motivating, varied, fun and gets results. *Cardio Kickboxing*® fits the bill.

It is what has worked for me for over nearly four decades. Occasionally, I do some running, biking, or lifting weights but my main method of staying healthy and fit has always been boxing or kickboxing workouts. It is not a cure for cancer, but it may prevent you from getting heart disease. It is what works for me and thousands of other fitness kickboxing enthusiasts. I am sure that it will work for you!

The Final Word. Perhaps you are thinking *Cardio Kickboxing*® is just a trend?

The advent of *Cardio Kickboxing*® workouts during the last decade has, in some fashion, benefited the following industries:

1. Health clubs are able to offer an effective fitness program that is an exciting alternative to conventional aerobics classes. There was and always will be programming options such as the slide, pilates, group cycling, yoga, boot camp, and fire drill classes. How much longevity they have is another issue. Martial arts-oriented fitness classes, especially those that utilize equipment, bring more men into the group fitness setting. For those women who want more sports rather than dance oriented classes, they are a sure-fire hit.

2. Many martial arts schools now offer these classes in conjunction with their regular class schedules whether it be Karate, Tae Kwon Do, Kung-Fu, or Ju-Jitsu. Most classes are full in the evening. This program helps generate additional revenue especially in the morning and during the noon hour when the school is rather quiet. These classes are also appealing to adults who do have not have the time or inclination to study for a black belt, but desire some sort of self-defense based activity.

3. Boxing gyms in the past were frequently difficult to operate financially. Unless there was a successful stable of professional fighters, the gyms were generally run down. Most aspiring world champions were from lower economic backgrounds and could not afford to pay much in dues to help contribute to the rent or training equipment. Nowadays, many gyms are supported substantially by those paying for fitness boxing and kickboxing classes. They are not there necessarily to become as skilled or conditioned as a professional fighter, but they can certainly train like one. It is not uncommon to find gyms that offer boxing, kickboxing, Muay Thai, cardio boxing, and *Cardio Kickboxing*® classes seven days a week. They are all related activities.

4. The manufacturers of boxing and kickboxing equipment have seen the wisdom in developing and supplying equipment for the recreational user in addition to the competitive fighter. There are 26 million golfers in this country buying billions of dollars of equipment annually. Would it make sense for manufacturers to cater only to the hundred or so elite golfers? Everlast used to be *the* name for boxing equipment. Now there are dozens of companies out there making gloves, bags, focus mitts, and apparel; namely, Ringside, Century, TKO®, as well as numerous foreign equipment manufacturers trying to tap into this market.

The martial arts and fitness based martial arts programs including *Cardio Kickboxing®* collectively provide millions of people with some form of exercise, discipline, and self-improvement. The training can certainly be used for self-defense purposes under certain circumstances. However, we should be intellectually honest about believing that the acquired knowledge makes someone invincible. Confronting someone with a weapon, especially a gun (unless it is an absolute last resort), is not prudent no matter how much martial arts training you've had. Perhaps you recall the scene in the *Raiders of the Lost Ark* where Indiana Jones nonchalantly shoots one of his pursuers who was waving the sword? On a larger scale, without sounding facetious, if every single one of the 1.2 billion people in China were Kung-Fu or San Shou experts, it would not matter much against just a handful of nuclear weapons. This is, after all, the 21st century, not the feudal Far East.

Thus, it would follow that it is not necessary to view the traditional martial arts as anything much more than a physical art form, kickboxing as anything more than a sport or *Cardio Kickboxing®* as anything more than a fitness program—but they are what have worked for me.

Finally, I would recommend choosing an ominous sounding nickname for yourself and pretend to be a world-class fighter when you are working out. Maybe even have your name embroidered on your workout shorts. Have fun with it, take it to whatever level you wish. But, above all else, at least give *Cardio Kickboxing®* a try.

Cardio Kickboxing® is what it says it is...

- It is kickboxing.
- It is kickboxing for fitness.
- It is kickboxing for fitness in a circuit training format.
- It is kickboxing for fitness in a circuit training format using equipment.
- It is kickboxing for fitness in a circuit training format using equipment for *everybody.*

- It is *not* karate.
- It is *not* karate and aerobics.
- It is *not* karate and aerobics choreographed to music.
- It is *not* karate and aerobics choreographed to music on a step.
- It is *not* karate and aerobics choreographed to music on a step just for *hard-bodies.*

Frank Thiboutot
AKA "Sandpiper" (my "ominous" nickname derived from my skinny bird legs)

CHAPTER 1

The Sport of Kickboxing

Kickboxing is a ring sport very closely related to the sport of boxing. As a backdrop to this book, I will take you on a brief historical journey from the origins of the martial arts to the evolution of American kickboxing and, finally, to the evolution of kickboxing from a sport to a fitness program.

TRADITIONAL STYLES OF MARTIAL ARTS

Unlike most other sports, the skills that you learn and the skill you acquire as you practice kickboxing can also be used for self-defense purposes. This is because kickboxing is a sport that is rooted in martial arts traditions.

The martial arts encompass thousands of different styles and disciplines of fighting arts, most of which have their origins in the Far East. Many of these martial art systems can trace their roots back to the Shaolin Temples in China. The original temple was built in 495 A.D. northwest of Dengfeng County in Henan province. In 527 A.D. the Indian monk Bodhidharma, also known as Da Mo, arrived at the temple and initiated the Chan (Zen) sect of Buddhism there. Bodhidharma found these monks to be very weak physically and developed exercises that helped to make them healthier and stronger. The Shaolin priests further developed these exercises by replicating the fighting movements of animals. These exercises were used for self-defense as well as self-preservation. Initially, these techniques were handed down from generation to generation in secret, but over time they spread to other parts of China and neighboring countries thus, forming Shaolin kung fu and eventually the multitude of martial arts that are available for study today.

Most martial art systems include similar techniques, and these techniques can be slotted into four basic categories: strikes (with the hand), kicks, wrestling, and submission holds. The following is a simplified breakdown of what each category contains:

Hand Techniques	Kicking	Wrestling	Submission
punches	kicks	grabbing	grappling
open hand strikes	sweeps	tripping	joint locks
elbow strikes	knee strikes	takedowns	chokeholds

Differentiation between various martial art styles depends on the techniques that a particular style emphasizes, particularly in competition. For example, some systems of karate in addition to the punch with a closed fist emphasize open-hand and closed-fist striking techniques. The open-hand techniques include using the heel of the palm, striking the outer and inner edge of the hand, and so on.

Others styles, like Tae Kwon Do (TKD), emphasize kicking techniques. They use a number of kicks beyond the basic front and round-house kicks; TKD often include such kicks as side kicks, spinning side kicks, hook kicks, axe kicks, and wheel kicks. During training (but not usually in competition) they also practice jumping or flying kicks, kicks that are executed while jumping in the air. You must practice for years to execute flying kicks efficiently and effectively.

Unlike karate and TKD, Judo emphasizes wrestling, throws, and takedowns, and Jujitsu (which recently became popular with the introduction of Ultimate Fighting contests) emphasizes submission holds. Some arts place emphasis on a combination of techniques such as Thai boxing, which permits punching and kicking under its system of rules for competition. San Shou allows punching, kicking, and takedowns. Many of these martial art techniques were originally meant to be lethal, so they were modified for competition purposes to protect the fighters from severe or life threatening injuries.

Martial Arts in America. Two people stand out in my mind as the primary contributors to the initial martial arts education of Americans in the 1960s and 1970s. They are Ed Parker and Bruce Lee. Ed Parker is considered the Father of American Karate. He introduced American Kenpo, which is a martial arts system that is an adaptation of the classical Okinawan systems of karate. Grandmaster Parker, a native of Hawaii, first learned these arts from Professor William K.S. Chow who had introduced some modifications to the traditional system. Parker is credited with revolutionizing these martial arts concepts and skills even further to fit our modern needs.

In the late 1960s, Bruce Lee brought the Chinese martial arts to the public's attention with his portrayal of the character, Kato, on the weekly television *series The Green Hornet* and through his movies, *Fist of Fury* (1972), *The Way of the Dragon* (1972), and *Enter the Dragon* (1973). Bruce Lee also introduced the American public to his martial arts system Jeet Kune Do, or JKD as it is more commonly known. This style was also considered "no style" in that it combined the stronger points of western boxing, Thai boxing, Wing Chun, karate, and grappling; yet, it was not bound to the ritual and dogma of its traditional contemporaries.

FROM MARTIAL ARTS TO KICKBOXING

Karate was the first of the martial arts to become popular in the United States mainly because of America's occupation of Japan, Okinawa, and Korea after the wars. Many Americans became more aware of Asian martial arts as servicemen were stationed in Asia. They brought back knowledge of martial arts virtually unknown in the United States previously. As the interest in martial arts grew in the United States so did the interest in martial arts (primarily karate) tournaments where competitors could test their skills against each other. At the time, these tournaments focused on the art of karate. As the athletes competed at these tournaments, however, there was often controversy regarding the methodology of scoring the matches and determining the winners. This was especially true in the open tournaments because so many different styles were represented. This controversy revealed itself in each of the three types of competitions conducted at most of these tournaments:

1. **Forms competitions.** The Japanese term for forms is known as *kata*; the Koreans call these forms *hyungs*. They are stylized routines similar to a gymnast's floor routine. Competitors perform traditional sequences of punches, kicks, and blocks in varying degrees of difficulty. They usually simulate defensive scenarios against multiple attackers. Judges subjectively scored these forms; higher scores were awarded for style, authenticity, and focus.

2. **Weapons competitions.** Similar to the form competitions, participants perform stylized routines—only this time using various traditional weapons and simulating defensive maneuvers. Weapons include, but are not limited to, staffs, knives, Sai, and Nunchaku. These competitions were also subjectively judged.

3. **Sparring (point fighting) competitions.** Point fighting (sparring) was a more realistic application of the various martial arts techniques that were learned in the *dojo*, the Japanese term for karate school (*dojung* in Korean, *kwan* in Chinese). Judging these matches was somewhat less subjective than the forms or weapons competitions; unfortunately, even point fighting was not entirely objective. In the 1960s and 70s, however, there was difficulty in determining what was actually an effective point since the punch or kick was supposed

to stop short of the target. The fighter was supposed to demonstrate control over his techniques, and the judges relied on the fact that the competitor actually could have landed the blow effectively. The rules that were meant to protect the competitors diluted the objectivity of the decisions. Despite the rules, some fighters made more contact than was allowed, and some just disregarded the rules and were disqualified for making excessive contact. Point fighting further developed with the advent of safety gear in the form of foam foot and hand pads (created by Master Jhoon Rhee, considered the Father of American TKD). Thus, light-contact sparring competitions emerged in certain events.

Further complicating the scoring process of all three types of tournament competitions was the nationalistic tendencies of the various judges. The Chinese stylists did not often recognize Japanese karate as legitimate; the karate practitioners did not acknowledge the TKD competitors, and so on. Thus, the need arose for a more objective comprehensive scoring system for the competitors especially those who were competing in sparring matches.

AMERICAN KICKBOXING EMERGES

In 1974, the Professional Karate Association (PKA) sanctioned the first full-contact karate matches in the United States. These matches are now known as American, or North American, style kickboxing. The founders of the PKA, Don and Judy Quine, are credited with creating and building the sport here in the U.S. The PKA brought together various martial arts stylists to compete against each other in sparring under the same set of rules and regulations. Most of the early PKA competitors (Joe Lewis, Bill Wallace, Jeff Smith, Chuck Norris, and Joe Corley) were already competing as karate point fighters.

The rules that were established for kickboxing were based on the rules of boxing rather than those of point fighting. These rules are still pretty much the same today as they were then. Weight divisions were established, and the number of rounds ranged from three (for amateur fighters) to twelve (for professional, world title fights). The major and obvious difference between a boxing match and a kickboxing match was that the fighters were allowed to kick as well as punch. To prevent a kickboxing bout (also known as a full-contact bout) from reverting to a boxing match, a minimum kick requirement of eight kicks per round was required for professionals and six per round for amateurs. The objective, however, of both boxing and kickboxing remained the same: during the match the competitors' objective was to try to knockout or to win a decision by inflicting enough damage on the opponent. Decisions were based on points scored using a ten point "must" system. The must system worked as follows:

Each round, a score of ten points was awarded by each of the three judges to the winner of the round, and the opponent received a score of nine points or less. This system was still somewhat subjective, but this cumulative scoring system was a much fairer way of determining the winner.

Many martial arts instructors considered kickboxing—this hybrid of martial arts and boxing—to be blasphemous. These instructors were entrenched in traditional martial arts philosophy and believed that blocking, striking, and kicking should only be used:

1. With control when participating in point fighting tournaments
2. When absolutely necessary for self-defense purposes.

Thus, it was not easy to gain initial acceptance for kickboxing within the martial arts community.

Furthermore, the techniques learned to compete in the sport of kickboxing are very sport-specific as compared to traditional martial arts. Kickboxers—similar to western-style boxers—train to fight one opponent at a time, whereas traditional martial artists learn techniques that teach them to defend themselves against multiple attackers. Thus, the training methodologies are different for a kickboxer training to compete in a ring sport and for a traditional martial artist training for self-defense purposes. Examples of these differences include:

It is illegal in the sport of kickboxing to make contact with any part of the glove other than the padded portion covering the knuckles. Thus, all other use of the hand (inside the glove) such as a palm-heel strike or a knife-edge strike is considered a foul under the rules of the sport. Conversely, these strikes are fundamental martial arts techniques. Naturally, the choice of training methodologies depends on the strikes permitted in competition.

A martial artist may use a back kick to thwart an attacker behind him, but since there is no opponent standing behind a kickboxer in the ring, he does not need to practice that particular kick while training. He may opt to use what is known as a spinning sidekick, but frankly that kick is of secondary importance and is used only occasionally in the ring. The three primary kickboxing kicks are the front kick, the roundhouse kick and lead-leg sidekick. Further differentiation is seen in the sport of Muay Thai, also known as Thai Boxing, where the fighters seldom use any kick during a bout other than their soccer-style roundkick. Training for each of these disciplines obviously varies according to the kicks used in competition.

KICKBOXING VS. MUAY THAI

Muay Thai has a history dating back to ancient times in Thailand. It has its own set of rules and regulations similar to, but not the same as, American kickboxing. Because of warfare with the Chinese, Mongols, and Burmese, the Thai people first developed this art for battle and self-preservation. The techniques of this art were passed on through a manual of warfare known as the *Chupasart*. Muay Thai originally utilized knives, spears, battleaxes, and swords as well as the "eight limbs," including the two hands, two elbows, two feet, and two knees. Some people include the forehead as the ninth limb.

As an adaptation of the military arts, Thai boxing then became a popular ring sport in Thailand the 1920s and has since become the national sport of Thailand. It is commonly referred to there as "the sport of kings". Thai boxers train at numerous regional training camps. The fighters in these camps lead a very spartan existence compared to the standards for athletes in the United States. They train at an early age competing at various local fairs and venues in hopes of someday competing at one of the two major stadiums in Bangkok. The titles that are coveted most by the Thai fighters are the championship belts awarded at the Lumphini and Rajadamnern stadiums. Their training existence is literally, "the survival of the fittest." In Thailand, Muay Thai champions are considered heroes. The sport is so popular that it is seen regularly on TV four to five times a week. Many former champions and fighters have immigrated to other countries to help spread this sport worldwide. Muay Thai is gaining popularity and stature in Europe (especially in Holland and France), Australia, and Japan. It is now in direct competition in North America with American kickboxing.

Several distinctions between Muay Thai and American kickboxing exist. For example, Muay Thai is noted for its use of the shins rather than the instep of the foot when executing a roundhouse kick. American kickboxing employs the instep. Additionally, Muay Thai rules legally allow the use of debilitating elbow and knee strikes, making Muay Thai the most dominant of the ring sports when compared to conventional boxing and American kickboxing. American kickboxing and the PKA made the use of elbows and knees illegal and required fighters to wear foam shin guards as well as the aforementioned footpads. This was done as a means to protect the fighters from serious injury (much like the boxing glove is used in boxing matches) rather than fighting with bare knuckles. By modifying the amount of damage that could occur during the bout and reducing the amount of risk taken, the sport was made more appealing for the competitors. Such changes were made because it was felt that all-out brutal combat in the ring would not be acceptable to the American public as a sport. In short, the fans ultimately determined the acceptability of the sport in this country; the development of the PKA rules considered the American public's desire for a more sports-like, less brutal competition. This consideration for audience needs is not unusual in the development of emerging sports. For example, Americans' preference for kickboxing rather than Muay Thai can be likened to the preference Americans have for football over rugby. The British, of course, prefer rugby to football. They understand it and are familiar with it because they grew up playing it. The same can be said for preferences that audiences have for either kickboxing or Muay Thai.

THE GROWTH OF AMERICAN KICKBOXING

As you can see, the evolutionary process from competition in martial arts tournaments to PKA (kickboxing) tournaments was somewhat of a "re-invention of the wheel" since the similar ring sport of Muay Thai already existed. However, since we occupied Japan and not Thailand after World War II, karate rather than Muay Thai became the dominant martial art in this country since the sixties, and, thus, the sport of kickboxing took somewhat of a circuitous route to develop in the U.S.

In the 25 plus years since the inception of the PKA, the sport of kickboxing has gained attention worldwide. It first started to receive recognition in the early eighties when it was seen regularly on the fledgling ESPN network. As early on as 1976, Howard Hanson and Arnold Urquidez founded the World Karate Association (WKA), and the PKA began receiving competition from other sanctioned organizations. Other sanctioning bodies had a hand in helping to popularize the sport of kickboxing. These organizations include: KICK (Karate International Council of Kickboxing), PKC (Professional Karate Council), FFKA (Full Force Karate Association), PKF (Professional Karate Federation), IKBF (International Kick Boxing Federation), WAKO (World Association of Kickboxing Organization), and USKBA (U.S. Kick Boxing Association). Additionally, in the late nineties and early into the new century, the aforementioned WKA, the ISKA (International Sport Karate Association) and the IKF (International Kickboxing Federation) were the three largest and most far reaching sanctioning bodies in the sport of kickboxing worldwide. The popularity of the sport and the increase in governing bodies for it was no different than what has occurred in the sport of boxing with the various sanctioning bodies governing that particular sport.

ENTER FITNESS KICKBOXING

The more recent arrival of a variety of fitness kickboxing programs, in general, brought some confusion as to the actual definition of kickboxing. However, it also brought a dramatic increase in the amount of attention given to the sport of kickboxing since gyms have begun to offer fitness boxing and fitness kickboxing classes (as have health clubs and martial arts schools). These new programs enabled gym owners to generate more revenue and more revenue translates into cleaner facilities with better equipment and an increase in the attractiveness of kickboxing/fitness kickboxing to the general public. In fact, many women, accustomed to the atmosphere in a martial arts school or health club, are now training alongside of the amateur and professional fighters in boxing/kickboxing gyms. In the past, they rarely ventured into these places. Naturally, this integration increased the fan base for the sport of kickboxing. Such was the original mission of the *Cardio Kickboxing®* program discussed in the preface and in the next chapter.

TRAINING AND COMPETITION

A key result of the development of the different kickboxing organizations is that there are now five basic systems of rules under which kickboxers can compete:

- Full-contact karate, which requires kicks to be thrown above the waist
- Freestyle rules, which permits kicks to the legs, but above the knee
- Oriental rules, which permits kicks to the legs as well as knee strikes to the body
- Thai-style rules, which permits kicks, knee and elbow strikes to any part of the body
- San Shou rules, which permits kicks to the legs, but which also awards additional points for takedowns.

These days, a complete kickboxer may be defined as one who practices all ring sports, much like a complete martial artist will learn the four major components of martial arts (i.e., striking, kicking, wrestling, and submission holds). That way, as a competitive fighter, he or she can also gain more ring experience and remain more active by switching from boxing to kickboxing to Muay Thai bouts depending on what bouts the manager or promoter has available. For example, Troy Dorsey became the ISKA world champion in kickboxing as well as the IBF world champion in boxing. For those readers who would like to be able to further differentiate one kickboxing competition from another, please refer to Appendix, Rules and Regulations Overview.

This cross-competition helped bring legitimacy to kickboxers within the boxing community itself. As previously mentioned, kickboxers in the late seventies and early eighties not only had hard time being accepted by the traditional martial artists, but weren't highly regarded by the boxing community either. Since they were initially trained as point fighters, for the most part, boxing experts thought they could not box very well. (The counter argument was that boxers did not kick very well either).

Now that has changed dramatically and kickboxing is more accepted than ever. Many kickboxers do not even have backgrounds as traditional martial artists. Right from the start, they cross-train in boxing, kickboxing, and Muay Thai techniques. The alliance between the sports of boxing with kickboxing now seems stronger than the former alliance of traditional martial arts with kickboxing.

This is apparent in the kickboxers' training facilities. Although some may still train at martial arts schools, for the most part, kickboxers frequently train in gyms that offer boxing.

Regardless of where they train, kickboxers incorporate varying degrees of the following components necessary to improve their athletic performance. Other words can be used to describe them, but they are categorized as the five 'S'es to more easily recall them:

Skill   Speed   Stamina   Strength   Psyche

These terms are often confused with those that are needed to improve either one's health or fitness levels: cardiorespiratory fitness, muscular strength and endurance, body composition, and flexibility.

All athletes must develop and constantly work on all of the above mentioned five 'S'es to achieve success against the competition. The higher the level of competition, the more the need for refinement, practice, and conditioning. Sport by its nature has a tendency to dictate those areas on which an athlete must focus to improve. This is true of both individual and team sports. For example, I believe that golf is an individual sport that requires a very refined level of skill as well as a strong mental frame of mind (psyche). Stamina and strength, though important, are secondary factors in becoming a better golfer. A sprinter, on the other hand, needs speed, stamina, and strength to be successful with skill being less significant, but still necessary, to his overall success. Within a team sport such as football, I think that a lineman needs more strength than skill and the quarterback relies more on skill than strength.

It would be safe to say that in the sport of kickboxing, you would need to work on all five components, particularly to achieve success on a world class level. No matter how great your skill level, for instance, it would break down during the course of an actual bout without a great degree of stamina. It would goes without saying that you had better be physically prepared as well as have a strong mind once you step into the ring to face a high-performing opponent who believes he or she has the superior skill, speed, strength, stamina, and mental toughness to take you on.

Though it is a bit beyond the scope of this book because it is not required as part of a fitness program, full-contact sparring with protective equipment is, I believe, the only way to determine whether or not the kickboxing skills you learned are truly ingrained, polished, and effective. Those athletes who want to compete as fighters usually train in additional sessions specific to sparring. For more insight on the behind-the-scenes activity that takes place for a fighter to climb into the ring, see www.ringside.com, click on kickboxing, and read the article in the archives on "U.S. Team Competes in Mainland China."

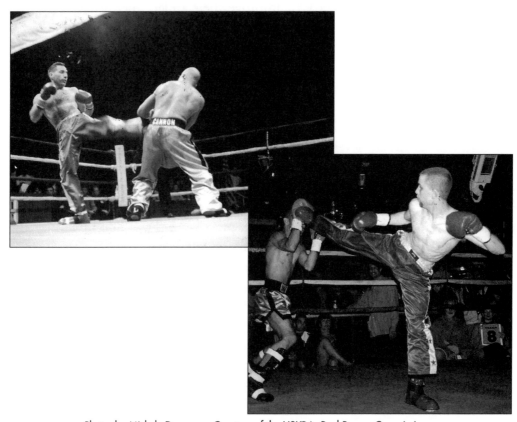

Photos by Michele Degamon, Courtesy of the USKBA, Paul Rosner Commissioner

CHAPTER 2

Cardio Kickboxing®

"Fitness club members are hearing and heeding the call of martial arts workouts, which are quickly becoming what step aerobics was to the early 1990s. Participation rates in martial arts exercise are so high that the demand is sur-passing that of some of the most firmly entrenched group exercise formats of this decade."

—ACSM's Health and Fitness Journal, *December 1999*

Having witnessed many training systems practiced by martial artists, boxers, and kickboxers over the years, I have found several things to be evident:

- Most traditional martial arts styles were passed down from instructor to instructor with the teaching methodologies being very similar within a particular style, but not necessarily similar from style to style.

- There appeared to be no specific clear-cut system or plan to train a boxer or kickboxer. The training methodologies varied from trainer to trainer since most boxers and kickboxers did their training alone (except when sparring), not in a group setting.

Thus, it was evident to train a large group of martial artists who aspired to become kickboxers there was a need to have a specific format for them to follow.

If they already had the basic skills, they needed to polish them until they were so ingrained that the basics became natural. For those just starting out, they needed a routine to practice kickboxing techniques that were effective in the ring, not martial art skills needed for self-defense.

In any event, both the seasoned as well as inexperienced kickboxers needed to systematically do sport-specific warm-up drills that covered footwork, bobbing and weaving, a review of their basic punches and punching combinations followed by a review of the basic kicks and kicking combinations. They then needed to blend their punches and kicks together in combinations. From there, they should work on the various pieces of boxing and kickboxing equipment on a round by round basis replicating an actual bout. Afterward, they would do some strength-ening and conditioning drills such as plyometrics or skipping rope combined with push-ups and crunches. To cool down, they would stretch. This was my particular general format for training a fighter, but it was also the genesis for the original *Cardio Kickboxing*® program that was to be promoted to the fitness industry.

Cardio Kickboxing® was created in the early 1990s to promote awareness of the sport of kickboxing to the general public. The idea was that an exciting, high-action fitness routine incorporating the workout of a kickboxer would appeal to a significant public audience and, therefore, promoting the wider acceptance of the sport of kickboxing. Furthermore, you will see that *Cardio Kickboxing*® is based on sound principles of exercise science making it the most exciting and effective fitness program on the market. In addition to helping promote the sport of kickboxing, *Cardio Kickboxing*® provided an alternative workout to conventional aerobic classes.

The *Cardio Kickboxing*® workout had been modified somewhat from time to time in accordance with established fitness industry protocol. For example, *Cardio Kickboxing*® instructors no longer rotate their heads in full circles to loosen up their necks or extend their knee beyond the top of their foot to stretch the hamstrings when teaching a class. These are warm-up procedures that fighters have done for years past, but are considered contraindicated and "unsafe" within the fitness industry. There is always going to be some compromise on methodology when it pertains to exercise programs for the general population, but the fundamentals of boxing and the kicking techniques found in the martial arts, specifically in kickboxing, remain the core drivers of the *Cardio Kickboxing*® program.

There may be variations on what types of kicks you use or emphasize while training or in an actual bout, but it is safe to say that kickboxing can generally be defined as boxing with basic kicking added. As with punching, learning to kick in the air is just the first step in the process. You then must apply these punches and kicks to a target such as a heavy bag, punch mitts, or kicking shield. The final step is to try to effectively apply these kicks to a sparring opponent or an attacker in a self-defense situation. You will quickly realize that there are other factors to consider beyond the skill and conditioning required in these situations. Some of the factors include gauging distance, being able to make contact to the more vulnerable areas of the body, reacting to and controlling a rush of adrenaline when working with a partner and so on. In summary, however, by combining the footwork and punching ability of a boxer with the kicking skills of a martial artist, you will have the basics required for the sport of kickboxing.

Contrary to popular belief, the most important aspect about learning boxing is the footwork. Being able *to punch* is one thing, being able *to box* is another. Initially learning the various basic punches followed by punching combinations are obviously important, but you first have to move into position to punch in order to punch *effectively*. Secondly, you also need to avoid getting punched back as much as possible. Learning to move your feet like a boxer can also be a valuable skill in a self-defense situation, but with regards to the *Cardio Kickboxing®* workout, the more you move your feet and use the major muscles of the legs, the better the workout *you will* receive.

This same line of thinking applies to kicking. It is one thing to learn a specific kick. Effectively executing and landing that kick on a target with speed and power is another matter all together. The martial art of Tae Kwon Do, for example, teaches you not only to kick, but to be able kick a moving target, namely an opponent who is also constantly moving to avoid getting kicked. Conditioning plays an important role in being able to do this for any length of time, particularly in competition.

Even though there has been some minor compromise on the methodology of presenting the workout of a kickboxer to general fitness enthusiasts, the fact remains that the format of the original program contains all the requirements for a fighter, but it also forms the basis for a sound fitness program.

The *Cardio Kickboxing®* workout contains the following five components that improve physical fitness and are essential to any fitness program:

- cardiorespiratory activity
- muscular strength training
- muscular endurance training
- flexibility training
- improvement in body fat composition.

GENERAL FITNESS GUIDELINES

Before discussing the actual program in detail, it is necessary to briefly understand some basic training guidelines for healthy adults. The quantity and quality of exercise needed to attain health-related benefits differ somewhat from what is recommended for fitness benefits. Many people continually confuse the amount of exercise needed to achieve health benefits, the amount of exercise needed for fitness benefits, or how much is necessary to achieve peak athletic performance. People who are usually inactive can improve their overall health by simply becoming even moderately active on a regular basis. Physical activity need not be strenuous to achieve health benefits. Furthermore, greater health benefits and/or fitness benefits can be achieved by increasing the amount of physical activity. The American College of Sports Medicine (ACSM) has summarized these guidelines for cardiovascular endurance as follows:

1. **Frequency.** Three to five days per week. Most fitness experts agree that exercising three times a week is necessary for maintaining fitness and weight control. The amount of improvement plateaus after three times per week and no apparent improvement occurs when exercising more than five times per week.

2. **Intensity.** 55% to 90% of your maximum heart rate. In order to optimize your cardiofitness, it is important to exercise at 55–90% of your maximum heart rate.

   The less fit or de-conditioned population should work more toward the lower ranges between 55–64%.

   Your maximum heart rate is calculated by subtracting your age from 220 and multiplying that number by 55/65–90% to obtain your training heart rate range.

   Example:
   $$(220–50 \text{ years}) \times 55\% = \textbf{93 } \mathbf{HR_{min}}$$
   and
   $$(220–50 \text{ years}) \times 90\% = \textbf{153 } \mathbf{HR_{max}}$$

   Thus, in this example, training range is between 93 and 153 bpm.

   Group fitness classes are generally broken down into beginner, intermediate, and advanced sessions. When multi-level participants are in the same class, optional lower intensity movements should be offered. In a *Cardio Kickboxing*® class, this is accomplished at the various stations of equipment where you are able to work out at your own skill and intensity levels.

   Intensity is closely related to the duration of an exercise as mentioned below.

3. **Duration.** 20–60 minutes of continuous aerobic activity. Duration, however, is dependent on the intensity of the activity. Exercising at a low to moderate intensity for longer periods of time is recommended for non-athletic adults. If you increase the intensity, the duration may have to be decreased until your fitness level improves and your body is able to adapt to the stress placed upon it. The delicate act of balancing intensity and duration is dependent on your fitness goals.

4. **Mode of activity.** Any activity that uses the large muscle groups continuously. A workout that exercises all of the large muscle groups will be more effective in improving fitness than those that focus on only one or two muscle groups. For example, you certainly get your heart pumping and use the larger muscles in the legs in a Spinning® class. However, you are not necessarily working out in a fashion that encompasses your total body. Therefore, kickboxing, which uses all the muscles in the upper and lower body, is a more effective fitness program.

5. **Resistance Training.** Strength training such as the use of free weights or Nautilus equipment is more commonly used in a health club environment. Bag work, i.e., punching and kicking a heavy bag can also provide resistance training. Fitness experts agree that for achieving the best overall fitness results, you need to do both a cardiovascular workout as well as a resistance-training workout. Resistance training tones and/or builds muscle, which is in itself a fitness benefit. In addition, muscle mass burns fat, and so further tones your body and improves your health. A *Cardio Kickboxing*® class combines aerobic with resistance training all in the same session.

Unfortunately, because of supermarket tabloids or TV infomercials, far too many people are concerned with how much they weigh rather than paying attention to the ratio of fat weight vs. fat-free weight. Fat-free weight refers to lean body mass, i.e., bone, muscle, organ tissue, water, and everything else. A 6'1" professional athlete may weigh 240 lbs. with a body fat percentage of 6%. Conversely, a non-athletic 6'1" male could also weigh 240 lbs. with a body fat percentage of 32%. They both weigh the same. Which person is likely to be healthier? Which person is likely to be more fit?

General Body Fat Ratios
(Source: American Council on Exercise)

	Women	Men
Essential Fat	10–12%	2–4%
Athletes	14–20%	6–13%
Fitness	21–24%	14–17%
Acceptable	25–31%	18–25%
Obese	32%+	25%+

BENEFITS OF CARDIO KICKBOXING®

Here we will explore is some detail eight important benefits the *Cardio Kickboxing*® workout offers.

1. *Cardio Kickboxing*® **combines both aerobic and anaerobic workouts.** The workouts that provide your body with maximum results are those that combine both aerobic and anaerobic properties. Aerobic activities are those that help stimulate the flow of blood and oxygen through the heart. An aerobic workout includes activities such as running, stair climbing, skipping rope, stationary bicycling, etc. An anaerobic workout consists of high intensity/short duration activities such as lifting weights, Nautilus, calisthenics, sprinting, etc. If you run exclusively, for example, you would benefit more if you chose to run a little bit less and add some weight training several times per week to your workout. Conversely, if you like to focus on lifting weights, your muscles will be more pronounced and you will have more definition if you add some running or stair climbing. Combining aerobic and anaerobic activity adds dimension and variety to your workout. Additionally, cross training can reduce injuries due to boredom, carelessness, and overuse of the same joints and muscles.

   An additional benefit of combining aerobic and anaerobic exercise is shown in the following example. Men with love handles and some excess fat over their abdominal muscles sometimes attempt to do more crunches to reduce their midsections. This may actually increase the size of the waist if done without an aerobic component in the overall exercise program. Essentially, you are building the muscles under the fat without proportionately reducing the amount of fat. Everyone has abdominal muscles. Some are more developed than others are, but in order to achieve the coveted washboard effect, the excess fat covering them up must be reduced so that the abdominal muscles can be seen. *Cardio Kickboxing*® provides you with an excellent proportion of both aerobic and anaerobic activity to keep your body in proper balance.

2. *Cardio Kickboxing*® **provides total-body exercise.** The workout that trains your entire body, not just specific body parts, provides you with the best overall fitness. Following is an example of the effects of total-body training.

   Women generally complain the most about their hips and thighs. Conventional wisdom advises them to do squats and lunges. That will certainly tone up the muscles in that area. However, in conjunction with an aerobic component and a total body workout, you can decrease the fat in all parts of your body, tone the muscles, and even build muscle in your upper body to be proportional to your newly fit thighs and buttocks. Simply stated, there is no such thing as "spot reducing." Otherwise, as Covert Bailey, the renowned fitness and nutrition expert has stated, "People who chew gum would have skinny faces." *Cardio Kickboxing*® works your entire body.

3. *Cardio Kickboxing*® **makes efficient use of time.** In a week there are 168 available hours. All you need is three hours of that time for a *Cardio Kickboxing*® workout. This is approximately 1.8 percent of your total time. If you count travel time to a health club, martial arts school, or boxing/kickboxing gym, it may bump that number up to maybe 4 percent but that still leaves you with 96 percent of your time to pay attention to everything else in your life. This is something to which you need to give serious consideration. The incorporation of exercise into your lifestyle will have immediate as well as long lasting benefits. In the scheme of things, *Cardio Kickboxing*® takes minimal time but provides maximum results.

4. *Cardio Kickboxing*® **provides valuable self-defense skills.** It is true that in order to put these skills to the real test you need to apply them to real targets rather than just practice the movements in the air. Using heavy bags, speed bags, and other equipment, you actually "land" your kicks and strikes. Additionally, the techniques taught in this program are actual precise techniques, not watered down imitations. Continued practice of these techniques will give you the solid foundation needed to use them on opponents. With *Cardio Kickboxing*®, you will become confident of your ability to understand and apply the self-defense techniques associated with this program.

5. *Cardio Kickboxing*® **boosts confidence and self-esteem.** Exercise helps you feel and look better physically. Generally speaking, when you feel and look better, your confidence level increases. The confidence that you gain through exercise can often transfer over into your social life and even to your profession. The more comfortable you are with yourself, the more confidently you will be able to cope with whatever life has in store for you.

6. *Cardio Kickboxing*® **relieves stress.** Most of us experience a great deal of daily frustration and aggravation that leads to stress. Some people relieve stress by using drugs, drinking alcohol, or overeating; however, reducing stress in such a negative manner is only a temporary solution that will only lead to more stress in the long run. A more appropriate method is to relieve your frustration and aggravation through physical

activity. Exercise increases the amount of hormone-like chemicals known as endorphins, which are released into the body by the brain to relieve pain and even depression. Stress, however, produces enzymes that reduce your supply of endorphins. If you do not exercise to stimulate that supply of endorphins, you are simply not feeling as well as you could feel.

Additionally, the *Cardio Kickboxing®* workout helps to relieve all your pent up frustrations by punching and kicking a heavy bag, for instance, rather than taking out your aggravations on some innocent person who may not even be the source of your tension.

7. **Cardio Kickboxing® increases energy levels and improves productivity.** Generally speaking, exercise boosts your energy levels. The more energy you have the more productive you become. Increased energy and productivity will not just remain in the gym; it will carry over into you personal and professional life as well. You will have greater stamina to get the job done, and you will have the energy to give your family the quality time they deserve.

Many times when you make the decision to get into shape, you attack this process too aggressively and consequently burn out. You may work out too hard and not give your body enough time to rest and recuperate. In other words, you do too much too fast and then become discouraged. It is wiser to gradually increase the frequency, the level of intensity, and the duration of your workouts. The circuit-training format of this program is designed to allow you to work out at your own pace. *Cardio Kickboxing®* can fit into you schedule in a way that helps to avoid burnout and gives you proper time to recover in between workouts so that your energy and productivity levels increase and stay that way.

8. *Cardio Kickboxing®* **is fun!** Unlike a traditional martial arts class, the music in this program will add to your stimulation and motivation. Unlike an aerobics class, the techniques that you learn in this program are numerous and challenging at all levels of fitness. Also, classes go by fast. Often there is so much going on that you do not even realize that you are working out. I have witnessed first-hand over the past eight years the expressions on people's faces when they are kickboxing for its fitness benefits. They remain intense and focused. They do not drift off and participate in a rote manner during the workout because there is so much happening that it demands their full attention. They really enjoy it!

ADDITIONAL BENEFITS

Although primarily designed for adults, the program can also provide benefits to adolescents as well. Student athletes can train in the off season with this workout to condition their bodies for their particular sport. Even at the high school level, sports are very competitive, and training in the off-season is a must to prepare for tryouts and the rigors of the next season. The boost in self-confidence that *Cardio Kickboxing*® provides can provide a mental edge when it comes to getting more playing time and performing well during actual game conditions.

For those students who choose not to play competitive sports, they surely need to exercise in some fashion. Exercise is important for everyone at all ages and should be fun and challenging to keep you interested. *Cardio Kickboxing*® certainly fits the bill!

POPULARITY OF FITNESS KICKBOXING PROGRAMS

It is common within the fitness industry to find that new programs come and go on a regular basis. This is because exercise requires discipline and is not always easy or convenient for some to incorporate into one's lifestyle. People who opt for the latest diet or trend that will work its magic overnight have missed the point all together. The *Cardio Kickboxing*® program as well as boxing or martial arts based fitness programs that followed it were accepted by the fitness industry in the mid-1990s because they were new and exciting, but also had substance.

Thomas "The Promise" Trebotich, the founder of *The Boxaerobic Exercise,* introduced cardioboxing workouts at about the same time as I introduced *Cardio Kickboxing*®. His format was choreographed to music similar to aerobics classes, but utilized some classic boxing equipment. A later edition of his program, *Kick Box Exercise*, added kicking techniques.

Sugar Ray Leonard's and Jill Goodacre's *Boxout* (1993) and Kathy Smith's and Michael Olajide's *Aerobox* (1994) videos also helped popularize boxing-for-fitness classes.

Since then, other hybrid kickboxing-for-fitness programs entered the market. Jim and John Graden's *Cardio Karate,* based in St. Petersburg, Florida, is sold mainly to martial arts schools who belong to National Association of Professional Martial Artists (NAPMA). This program is the best of the competing programs that utilize standard kickboxing equipment. Other non-equipment programs combine martial arts and aerobics, but not necessarily kickboxing.

- Marcus DeValentino's *Xtreme Cardio Kickboxing*
- Steve Doss's *Kardio Kickbox* (now known as *Power Kickbox-Ultimate Cardio*)

- Rodrigo Navarrete's *Funkicks*
- Bylle Dopps' *KickFit*
- Lisa Gaylord's *Cardio Combat*
- Janice Saffell's *Kickbox Express*
- Eversley Forte's *Cardio Athletic Kickbox*
- Aaron Lankford's *Power Kicks*

Even aerobic organizations are now certifying kickboxing instructors to teach classes. Generally speaking, however, such classes are usually considered too "dancey" to attract a significant male following. Additionally, the credibility of these classes among competitive boxers, kickboxers, and traditional martial artists is lacking. In any event, all of the above-mentioned programs have aided in the success of the *Tae-Bo* workout. *Tae-Bo* was formulated a number of years ago, but it only became popular on a large scale through the use of television infomercials beginning in the fall of 1998. Billy Blanks took his version of the martial arts/aerobics workout, which was already becoming more and more common in health clubs and martial arts schools, and introduced it to the home market. *Tae Bo,* however, should not be confused with the original *Cardio Kickboxing®* program

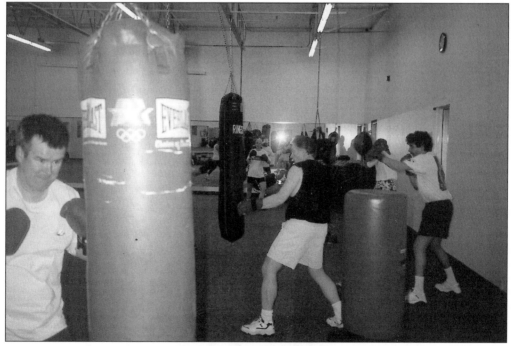

Figure 2-1. Class with equipment.

which was and always will be equipment intensive using authentic boxing and kickboxing techniques. This book offers an optional workout format in Chapter 8 for those health clubs or martial art schools who do not have the space or budget for classes utilizing equipment. However, they are grounded in the basics of kickboxing rather than some a mixture of aerobics with some martial arts techniques added to the class.

The attractiveness of one program over another is ultimately up to the practitioner. Aerobics-based programs, for example, string together various movements choreographed to music. This set up is very similar to martial-arts-based cardiofitness programs, which string together various martial arts techniques—or even mimic martial arts forms. In fact, most martial-arts-based fitness classes have a tendency to attract two primary audiences:

- Women especially aerobics enthusiasts familiar with patterns—the forms on which the programs are based are especially easy for women are accustomed to aerobics and dance-aerobics.

- Martial artists who prefer forms to point fighting and are, therefore, accustomed to training by repeating forms in a controlled environment.

Conversely, those programs that are based on boxing, Muay Thai, or kickboxing, like *Cardio Kickboxing*®, attracts boxers, kickboxers, women who are more sports- rather than aerobics-oriented, and martial artists who prefer point fighting.

Personally speaking, my own workouts will always consist of the use of equipment. I am not going to waste my time making up or practicing complicated patterns that would fit neatly and tidily into an aerobics setting.

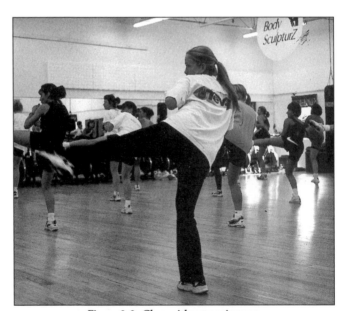

Figure 2-2. Class without equipment.

Furthermore, I am not going to pretend hitting a speed bag; I am going to practice hitting an actual speed bag. I am not going to pretend skipping rope; I am going to skip an actual jump rope. The reality that equipment brings to the workout offers the fitness benefits described earlier and the self-defense applications mentioned above.

Now that you have an understanding of what this program is, let us get started with the fundamentals!

CHAPTER 3

Fundamentals

We are now ready to get started. In kickboxing, it is not necessary to learn a lot of techniques, but rather to learn and practice the basics so that they become second nature. Initially, the focus will be on the techniques of American style kickboxing. The following fundamentals provide the foundation you need to later add on the intermediate and advanced techniques found in Chapters 6 and 7. The sport-specific techniques used in kickboxing are efficient and effective. They work in the ring as well as for self-defense. However, please note that whenever you see this icon, the offensive technique described is particularly effective for self-defense purposes.

HANDWRAPPING

Your hands (and feet) are your tools just like a mason uses a trowel to do his work. Give them as much protection as possible. To this end—and even though you have training gloves—wrapping the hands is necessary when you are ready to punch the bags. This added protection helps protect your wrists and the bones in your hands from injury upon impact. From the standpoint of mental preparation, I suggest that you wrap your hands even when you are doing a workout that does not use the bags. Wrapping the hands gives you a feeling that you are getting ready for a workout. It has a certain mental ambiance to it that is different from getting ready to go out for a run, for example. Additionally, your handwraps can also double as a sweat towel when they are not inside your gloves.

At first, the process of wrapping may seem time-consuming, but in a short time you will be able to wrap your hands quickly. To start, make sure the wraps are not are not too tight or too loose.

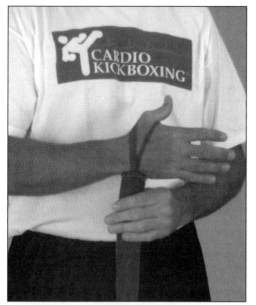

Figure 3-1

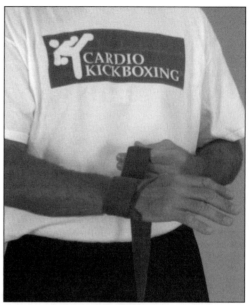

Figure 3-2

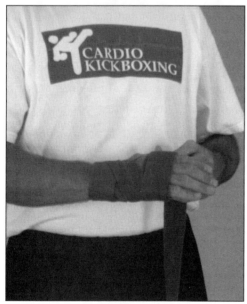

Figure 3-3

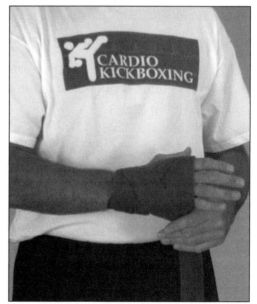

Figure 3-4

1. Start with the loop over the thumb. See Figure 3-1.

2. Wrap the cloth around the wrist several times. See Figure 3-2.

3. Wrap the cloth several times over the knuckles. See Figure 3-3.

4. Criss-cross the cloth to help prevent the wrist from bending. See Figure 3-4.

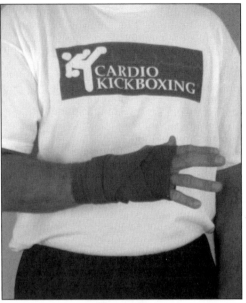

Figure 3-5

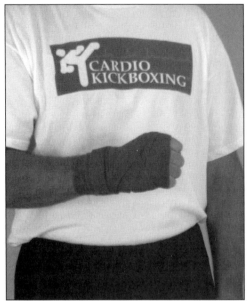

Figure 3-6

5. Tie the remainder off at the lower forearm. See Figure 3-5. There is no need to go between the fingers or around the thumb. Open and close your fist several times while wrapping to make sure it is comfortable. You do not need the extra long wraps; in fact, they may prevent you from closing your hand properly.

6. Figure 3-6 shows how the hand should look when finished.

The following fundamentals are presented from a right-handed perspective. For those who are left-handed, simply reverse the following terminology and techniques. For example, if you are right-handed, the right side of your body is considered the strong (power) side; if you are left-handed, the left side is your strong side. When right-handed, the left side is considered the lead (speed) side—and vice versa.

Also note that in the warm-up, you will sometimes be instructed to switch your lead side in order to balance the development of your muscles. When actually utilizing the punches and kicks, however, you do not switch stances and nearly always keep the lead foot in front.

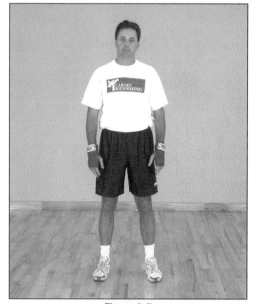

Figure 3-7

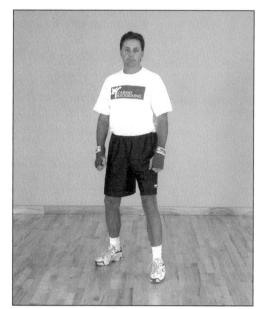

Figure 3-8

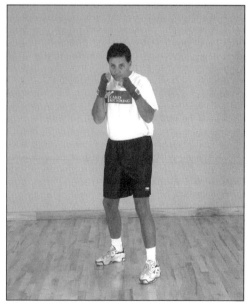

Figure 3-9

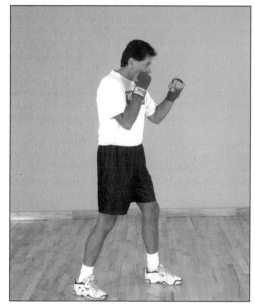

Figure 3-10

STANCE

1. Start with both feet parallel. See Figure 3-7.
2. Place the right foot back being careful not to be too wide, too narrow, or too deep. Keep your stance in a neutral boxer's/kickboxer's stance, not a rigid stance that you may use in traditional martial arts. To achieve this

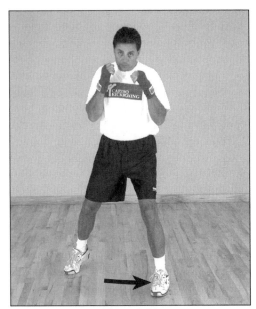

Figure 3-11

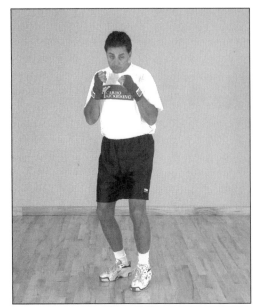

Figure 3-12

stance, keep your chest at a 45° angle rather than straight on to decrease your opponent's angle of attack. Always keep your hands up at cheek height with the left hand in the lead. This stance provides maximum mobility and balance. See Figure 3-8.

3. Hold your forearms close to your rib cage to protect your torso from body punches and from kicks above the waist. See Figures 3-9 (front view) 3-10 (side view).

FOOT MOVEMENT

The objective is to be able to move easily and comfortably in any direction. This is true from two perspectives. See Figure 3-11.

1. When competing against an opponent, the more you move, the less you tend to get hit—and the more easily you move into position to hit.

2. From a fitness perspective, the more you move, the better the workout.

It is essential never to cross your feet; the objective is to always slide. See Figure 3-12

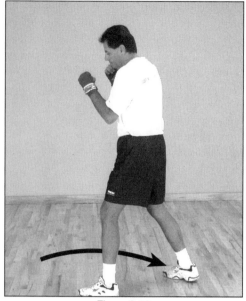

Figure 3-13

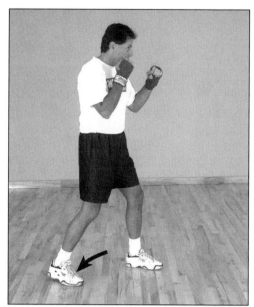

Figure 3-14

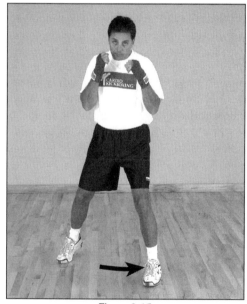

Figure 3-15

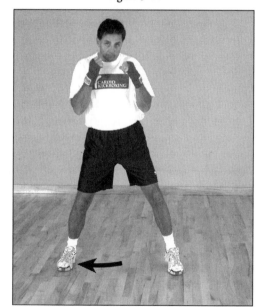

Figure 3-16

To start practicing, do the following:

1. Pivot left and right off the lead foot. See Figures 3-13 and 3-14.

2. Incorporate lateral movements by pushing off the foot to move in an opposite direction. See Figures 3-15 and 3-16.

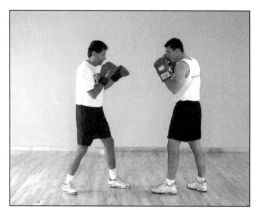

Figure 3-17

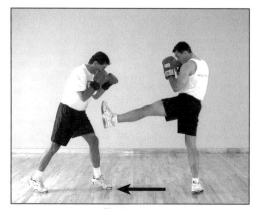

Figure 3-18

3. It is much easier to hit a stationary target rather than a target that moves. Learning to gauge distance is more important than any other attribute. If you can move in and out of position and be able to hit more and get hit less, you have the advantage. See Figures 3-17 and 3-18 for illustrations of moving in and out.

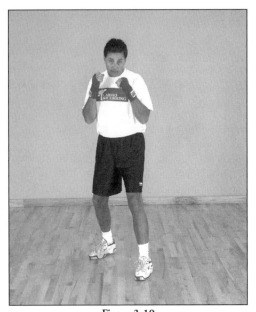

Figure 3-19

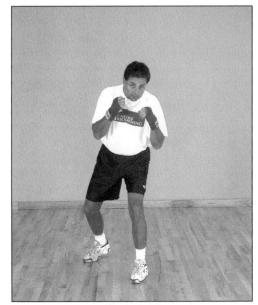

Figure 3-20

BOBBING AND WEAVING

In order to help you learn and remember the six directional options inherent in bobbing and weaving, the following instruction is presented as a sequence of six moves. When you learn the movements, your natural bob-and-weave movement will be more fluid—especially if you are actually competing against an opponent.

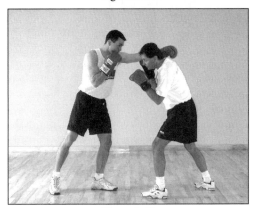

Figure 3-21

1. To start assume a neutral position and bend at the waist and knees. See Figure 3-19.

2. Move left at a 45° angle. See Figures 3-20 and 3-21. Move right at a 45° angle See Figure 3-22.

3. Move straight down (keep your eyes up). See Figure 3-23.

4. Lean back out of range. See Figure 3-24.

5. Weave left. Weave right. See Figure 3-25.

6. Return to the neutral position. See Figure 3-26.

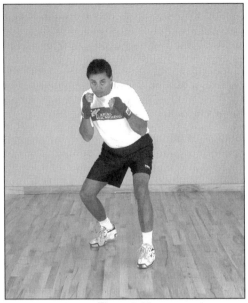

Figure 3-22

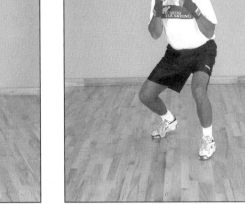

Figure 3-23

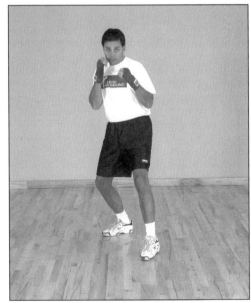

Figure 3-24

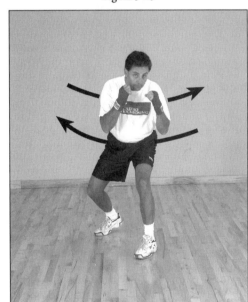

Figure 3-25

Later, you will bob and weave to slip an individual punch as it is coming at you without blinking or turning away from fear of getting hit. If someone is bigger and more powerful than you are, it does not matter if the punch misses you by an inch or a foot—as long as you slip it. (Remember, however, that if you spar or compete in the sport, you are going to get hit. It is not necessary to spar if you

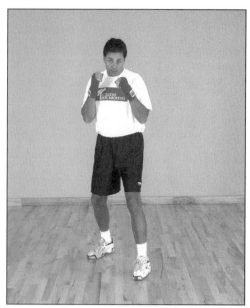

Figure 3-26

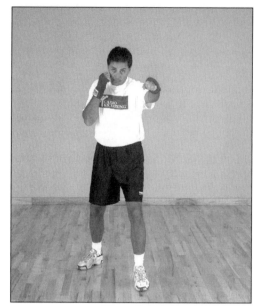

Figure 3-27

are doing this program solely to increase your fitness level, but if your goal is to take it to a higher level, contact is inevitable. Actual contact through sparring and competition is the only way to truly test your skills, to see how a punch or kick feels and how you react to actually being hit.)

For training purposes, you should be using a mirror to judge your reflection for feedback. You should visualize that the person in the mirror is your opponent who has the same height, weight, and experience level.

Four Basic Punches

If you are going to punch, you might as well punch hard. In competition, this is obvious. Yet, throwing a powerful punch also increases the effectiveness of your fitness workout. To do so, you must use the leverage from your legs to generate power. Just as a baseball player has to step into a pitch to hit the ball hard, a boxer or kickboxer must "step into" the punch. In actuality, you are really punching with your legs and hips; your fist is simply an extension of your legs. Also remember to keep the non-punching hand up at cheek level.

Jab

The jab is a speed punch thrown from the *outside* that is used to gauge distance from your opponent and set up other offensive techniques.

1. Start in a neutral position. Extend your left hand in a straight line toward the reflection of your chin (in a mirror). See Figures 3-27 and 3-28.

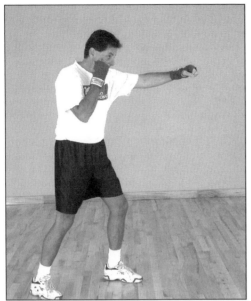

Figure 3-28

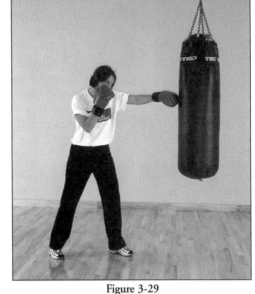

Figure 3-29

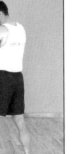

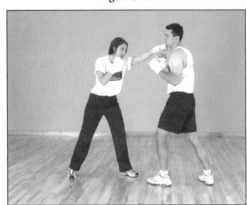

Figure 3-30

Figure 3-31

2. Twist the punch, so that when your arm is fully extended, your hand is palm down. As you extend your hand, take a three or four inch stutter-step toward your target with your lead foot. This action transfers your body weight toward the target. See Figures 3-29, 3-30, and 3-31.

3. When retracting your punch, bring it back in a straight line and back to your neutral hands-up position.

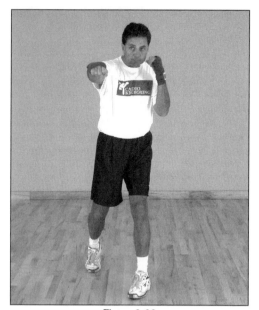

Figure 3-32

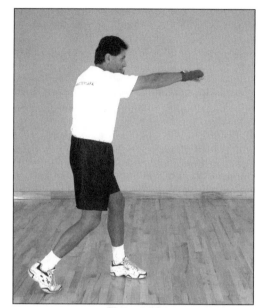

Figure 3-33

Cross

The cross is a power punch that takes longer to arrive at your target since it is further away than your jab. Both the jab and cross are distance punches usually thrown from the *outside*.

1. Start in a neutral position. Use your right hip with a push of the rear leg to initiate this punch, throw your cross directly toward the reflection of your chin (in a mirror). See Figures 3-32 and 3-33.

2. Also twist the arm so that when your arm is fully extended, your hand is palm down. See Figures 3-34, 3-35, and 3-36.

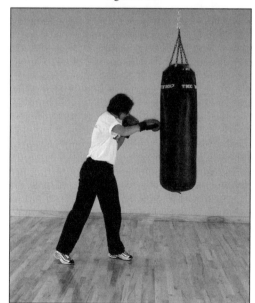

Figure 3-34

3. Maintain your balance and do not reach or allow your rear foot to leave the floor. You should come up on the ball of the foot, but if you leave the floor, you will negate the intended power of this punch.

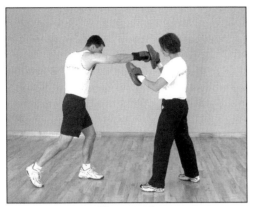

Figure 3-35

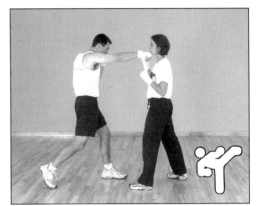

Figure 3-36

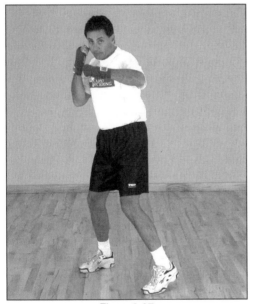

Figure 3-37

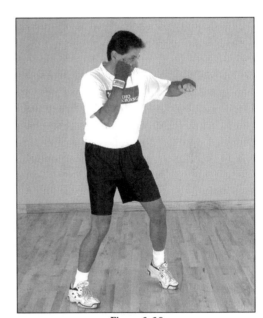

Figure 3-38

Hook

The hook is a tight, compact punch usually thrown on the *inside*.

1. Start in a neutral position. Initiate this punch by pivoting on the lead foot, which will bring your hip into play to increase power. See Figures 3-37 and 3-38.

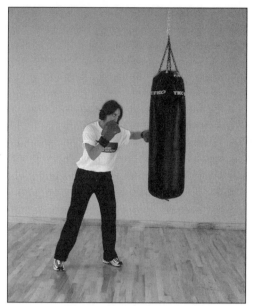

Figure 3-39

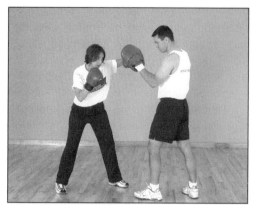

Figure 3-40

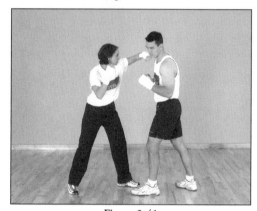

Figure 3-41

2. Extend your arm a circular fashion remaining close to parallel with the floor. Your fist can be palm-down or palm-in. The palm-down method uses more shoulder and lat muscles; the palm-in method uses more biceps. See Figures 3-39, 3-40, 3-41.

3. The target area is head level. To hook to the body, simply bend the knees first and execute the punch.

Uppercut

Similar to the hook, the uppercut is tight and compact and is usually thrown on the *inside*.

1. Start at a neutral position. To initiate this punch, first bend at the knees. The more bend, the more leverage you will gain. See Figures 3-42 and 3-43.

2. As you start to rise up, extend right hand upward almost perpendicular to the floor in front of your face. See Figure 3-44.

3. Unlike a cowboy's windmill punch in the movies, this punch uses a lot of hip and body action and is not a wide-angle punch. See Figures 3-45, 3-46, and 3-47.

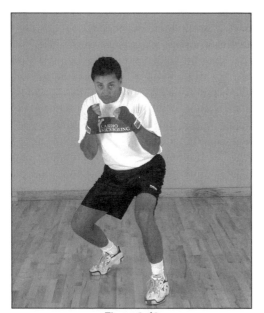

Figure 3-42

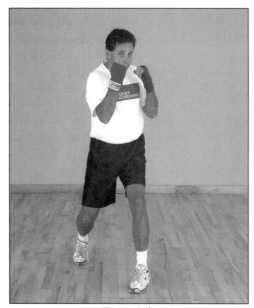

Figure 3-43

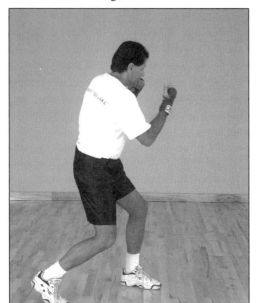

Figure 3-44

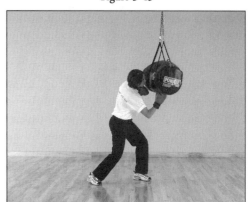

Figure 3-45

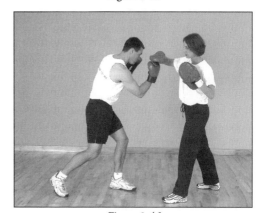

Figure 3-46

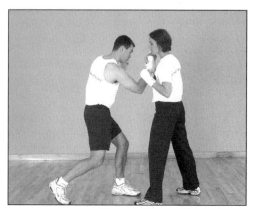

Figure 3-47

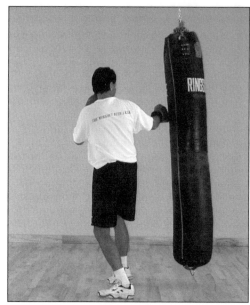

Figure 3-48

Spinning Backfist

This is another basic punch used in kickboxing, but is used very infrequently—most often as a counter-punch. The punch is thrown when your opponent starts toward you, and it lands as he or she closes the distance gap. This punch is illegal in boxing.

1. Assume a neutral position. Pivot clockwise on your lead foot 360°. It is very important that you start and finish in the same stance once the punch is completed.

2. As you begin to spin, raise your right fist to shoulder height with your elbow bent. Pick out your target over your right shoulder and strike with the back of the right fist. This is different than a martial arts backfist strike because it uses the momentum of the spin for greater power. See Figure 3-48.

Punching combinations are explained in detail in Chapter 5.

THREE BASIC KICKS

The three kicks described below—front kick, roundhouse kick, and lead leg sidekick—are used 90 to 95 percent of the time in kickboxing. There are, of course, other kicks such as the spinning sidekick, hook kick, and wheel kick, but they are not as efficient or expedient to use either in the sport of kickboxing or for self-defense. Please note that the front and roundhouse kicks are thrown from your natural kickboxer's stance.

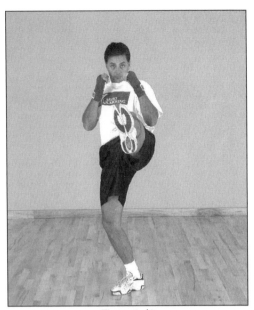

Figure 3-49

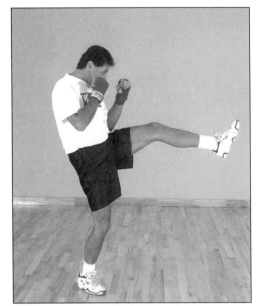

Figure 3-50

Front Kick

The use and execution of the front kick varies depending upon which leg kicks. A lead-leg front kick, like the jab, is executed quickly to set up other techniques and to gauge distance. A rear-leg front kick is similar to a cross punch in that it is a power strike, which takes longer to arrive at and travels further to the target.

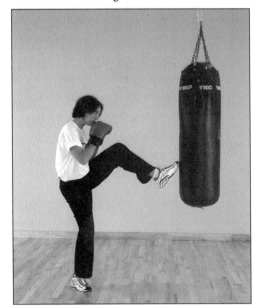

Figure 3-51

1. To execute using your lead leg, put your weight on your right leg and keep the knee slightly bent. Raise the left foot at the left knee as you snap the ball of your left foot mid-level into the air or against a heavy bag or kicking shield. Imagine your target to be the torso of your opponent. Be careful not to hyperextend or lock the knee. Then, return your foot to its normal position in your neutral kickboxer's stance. See Figures 3-49 and 3-50 for step-by-step illustrations of this kick. Figure 3-51 illustrates

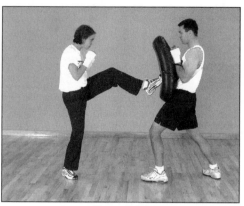

Figure 3-52

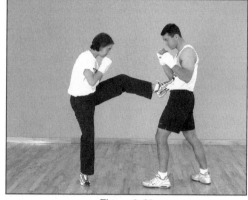

Figure 3-53

execution against the bag; 3-52 shows the kick against a kicking pad; Figure 3-53 against and opponent (or adversary).

2. To execute a front kick using your rear leg, raise you right knee and then thrust the ball of your right foot mid-level toward your target. Return your foot back to your normal stance. See Figures 3-54 and 3-55 for step-by-step illustrations of this kick. Figure 3-56 illustrates execution against the bag; 3-57 shows this kick against a kicking pad; Figure 3-58 against an opponent.

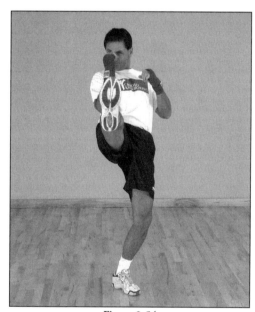

Figure 3-54

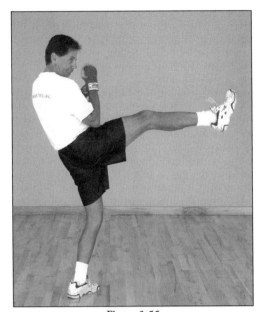

Figure 3-55

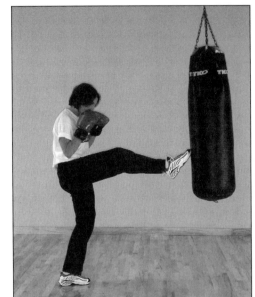

Figure 3-56

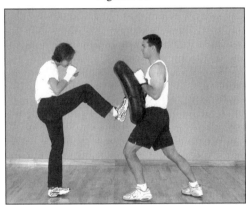
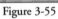

Figure 3-57

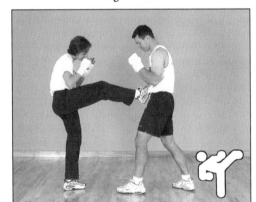

Figure 3-58

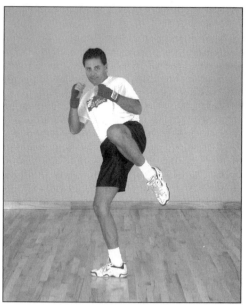

Figure 3-59

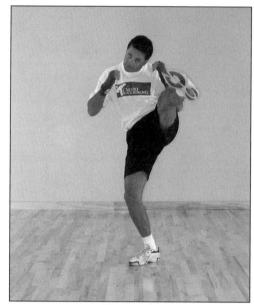

Figure 3-60

Roundhouse Kick

The roundhouse kick imitates a lead hook punch in its direction. Like the front and sidekicks, the roundhouse can be executed using either your lead leg or your rear leg.

1. To throw this kick using your lead leg, put your weight on your right leg and keep your knee slightly bent. Raise your left foot by the left knee and elevate the left hip. Slightly pivot on your right foot to attack from a 45–90 degree angle as you snap the top of your foot mid-level toward your target. Return your foot to its normal position. The angle of attack can either be a sharp angle (45°) or more rounded (90°) or somewhere in between. See Figures 3-59, 3-60, and 3-61 for step-by-step illustrations of this kick. Figure 3-62 illustrates execution against the bag; 3-63 shows the kick against a kicking pad; Figure 3-64 against an opponent.

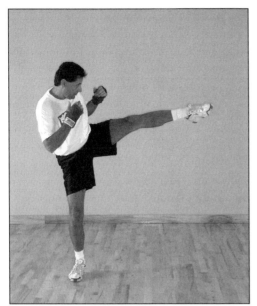

Figure 3-61

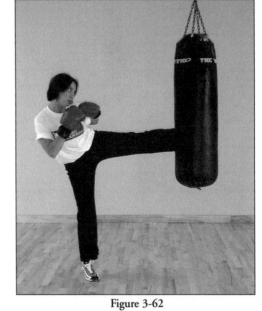

Figure 3-62

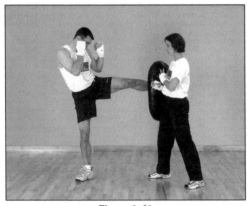

Figure 3-63

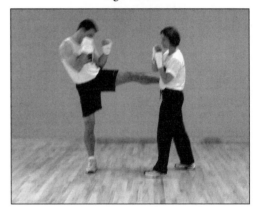

Figure 3-64

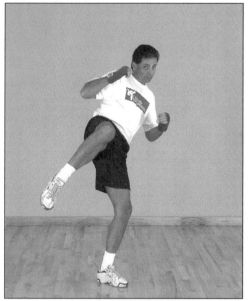

Figure 3-65

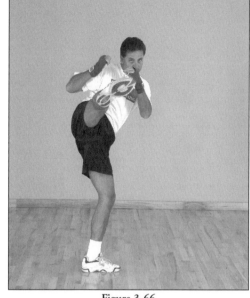

Figure 3-66

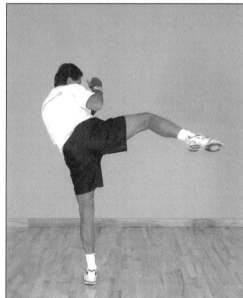

Figure 3-67

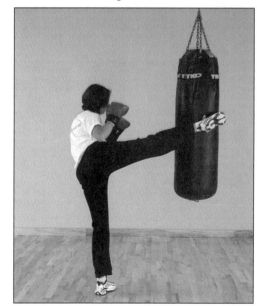
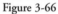

Figure 3-68

2. To execute this kick using your rear leg, raise your right knee elevating the right hip and while pivoting on the left foot thrust the top of your foot mid-level toward your target. Return your foot to its normal position. See Figure 3-65, 3-66, and 3-67 for step-by-step illustrations of this kick. Figure 3-68 illustrates execution against the bag; shows the kick 3-69 against a kicking pad; Figure 3-70 against an opponent.

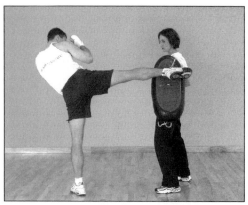

Figure 3-69

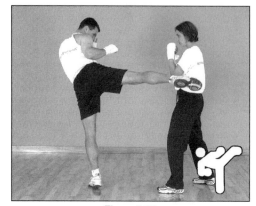

Figure 3-70

Sidekick

The sidekick is used as a counter-kick when your opponent starts toward you. In kickboxing, this kick is thrown using your lead leg only.

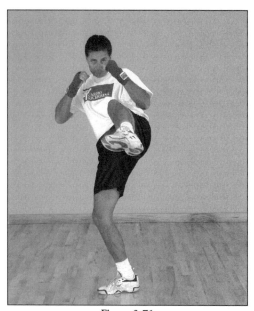

Figure 3-71

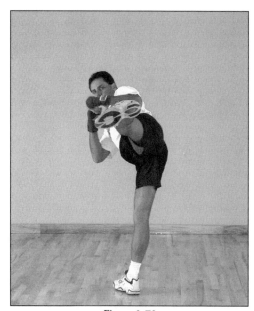

Figure 3-72

1. Put all of your weight on your right leg and pivot your right foot while shifting your chest so that you are facing the side. Allow your left hip to lead the kick. See Figure 3-71.

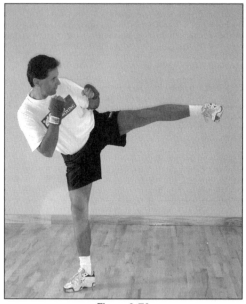

Figure 3-73

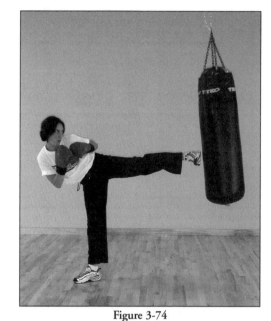

Figure 3-74

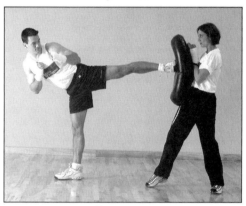

Figure 3-75

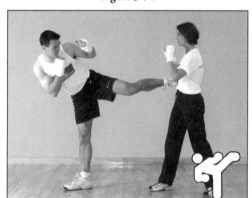

Figure 3-76

2. Extend your lead leg mid-level with your foot parallel to the floor. The point of contact is primarily the heel and bottom of your foot. See Figure 3-72 and 3-73.

3. Be sure to retract your kick using the quadriceps and then lower your foot to the floor. Shift back to your neutral stance. See Figures 3-74, 3-75, and 3-76.

Note: The kicks described in this chapter do not take into account the variations used by Muay Thai fighters who are allowed to kick below the waist to the legs and strike with the shin.

HELPFUL TIPS FOR KICKS

The following hints will help you practice proper structure and achieve the most effective kicks.

- To help overcome inertia for the lead leg in front and roundhouse kicks, it is easier to execute these kicks while in motion rather than standing still. The angle of attack is the main difference between kicks.

- With the roundhouse kicks, the point of contact is ideally the area from the middle of the instep to just above the ankle. Otherwise, you could hurt your ankle or knee. Also, be sure to be close enough when practicing on the bag so that you can wrap your foot around it as you would if you were kicking someone's waist by wrapping it with your instep. From a safety standpoint, it is better to be closer to the target than further away because if you err on the side of being too close, you will strike with your shin. If you are too far away, you will make contact more toward the toes—which will cause damage to you, not your opponent/bag.

- Try to retract your kicks as fast as you execute them to prevent them from being grabbed by your opponent.

- A single kick can be powerful. However, as fatigue sets (in a bout or when training), kicks have a tendency to diminish in speed and power They then have roughly the same force and effect as punches.

- For practice, you may want to change the level of your kicks: low, mid-level, and high. However, never try to kick high when competing or for self-defense purposes.

Please be aware that effective punching and kicking combinations are basic and simple. Once you become comfortable with them you can begin to add movement and more advanced combinations. One of the best ways to test their effectiveness is to pay attention to gap time. Just as there should be very little gap in time between punches thrown in combination, there should also be very little space between your punches and kicks. If there is too of a much gap, your combinations are too complex or may be martial-arts-oriented rather than kickboxing-oriented. Combinations with longer gap times give your opponent opportunities to strike in between your combinations. Punching and kicking combinations are discussed in detail in Chapter 5.

SHADOW BOXING AND KICKBOXING

You must learn and polish all your punches and kicks, but it is natural to have a tendency to rely on certain techniques over others. Actually, this preference in large part depends on your body type. For example, taller, leaner people will find it more comfortable to use the jab and cross. Shorter, more compact people will prefer to use the hook and uppercut.

If you prefer some of the basic kicks and punches, however, you tend to practice them more often than the ones you do not prefer. It is important when working out to give each strike equal attention. Think of it this way: the more weapons in your arsenal, the better the fighter. Knowledge is power.

Take care not to overdo the growth of your arsenal. In kickboxing, for example, it is generally more expedient to rely on basics and fundamentals and leave the fancy stuff for the movies.

To practice a shadowboxing or kickboxing workout, purchase a timer that can be set for two or three minutes of activity followed by a rest period of 15, 30, 45, or 60 seconds depending on your level of conditioning. Use the timer to simulate a bout. Train yourself to change your tempo and rhythm as you advance rather than just staying the same speed throughout each round.

Shadowboxing and kickboxing routines are discussed in more detail in Chapter 5.

BLOCKING

Unlike most martial art styles or systems, kickboxing does not utilize conventional blocks. While sparring or competing, it is unsafe to drop the hands to block because your opponent may be setting you up with a fake, thus causing you to drop your hand (to block) at the time when he or she actually punches. See Figures 3-77 and 3-78. In a self-defense situation on the street, your attacker might even break your hand or arm if you employed a traditional martial arts block.

In kickboxing, therefore, defensive tactics fall into three basic categories: foot movement, bobbing and weaving, and keeping your hands up and forearms close to your sides. These categories correspond to the following lines of defense:

1. The first line of defense in kickboxing is normally to move out of range especially, for a kick, hence, foot movement. See Figure 3-79.
2. The second is to move your head when you are in close. This is the effect of bobbing and weaving. See Figure 3-80.
3. The third is to actually absorb a punch on the gloves (see Figure 3-81) or a kick on the forearms (see Figure 3-82), thus the need for your hands and forearms to be in proper position.

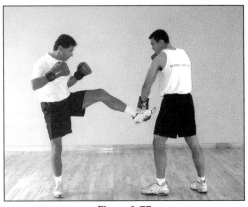

Figure 3-77

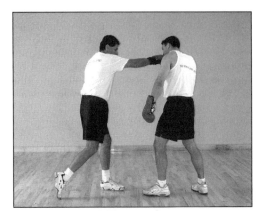

Figure 3-78

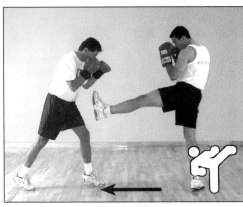

Figure 3-79

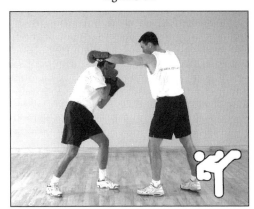

Figure 3-80

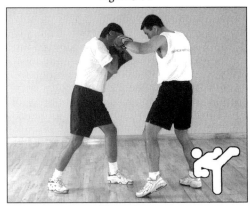

Figure 3-81

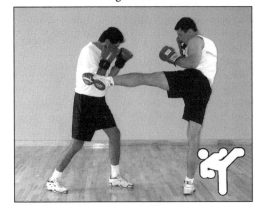

Figure 3-82

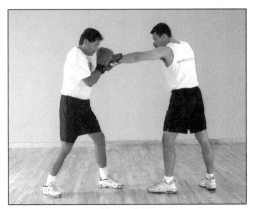

Figure 3-83

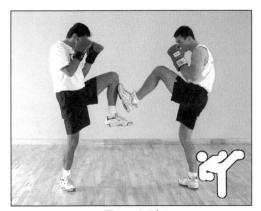

Figure 3-84

The parry, as shown in Figure 3-83, is occasionally employed with the right hand to deflect (not block) a jab. Additionally, in Thai boxing, you could block a kick to your legs by raising your knee and using your shin. See Figures 3-84 and 3-85.

Other than these few techniques, everything about kickboxing is offensively, not defensively, oriented. Therefore, as you and your opponents become more skilled and effective

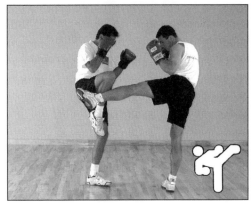

Figure 3-85

fighters, success becomes a "physical chess match" requiring strategy as well as pure physical ability.

If you are already performing some sort of cardiofitness kickboxing program at home or as part of a class, you may be already mimicking some of the techniques described in this chapter. It is important, however, to also understand their applications. For example, there is a knee raise and an arm pull down move done in many aerobics classes. It looks similar to a shin block, but these two moves are not the same. The shin block has a specific purpose as previously explained. Other than to perhaps work the hip flexor, this particular aerobics move does not have a specific purpose.

SKIPPING ROPE

Skipping (not jumping) rope is a great cardiovascular exercise that also improves coordination. This is not a high impact workout if you skip properly. To skip properly, your feet should leave the floor no more than an inch allowing

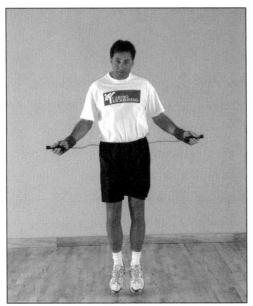

Figure 3-86

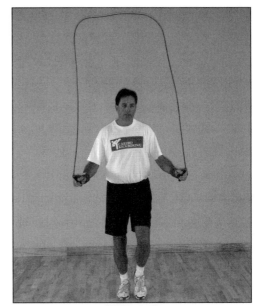

Figure 3-87

the rope to barely pass between the bottom of your athletic shoe and the floor. If you are new to this activity, first start without a rope to synchronize the timing of the hands and feet.

1. Start jumping with the feet together. See Figure 3-86.

2. Begin alternating left and right until you become familiar with the rhythm. See Figure 3-87. Be sure to keep your elbows close to your sides, otherwise, it will put too much stress on your shoulders. Your wrists do most of the work with regards to the speed of the rope. The faster your wrists turn, the faster the rope will move and the quicker you will have to pick up your feet.

This is the basic skip. Without learning it first, you will not be able to do some of the common "tricks" used to relieve boredom or bump up the intensity level. These more advanced moves include:

- Crosses (see Figure 3-88)
- Ski jumps (see Figure 3-89)
- Knee-ups (see Figure 3-90)
- Double jumps (see Figure 3-91)
- Squats (see Figure 3-92)

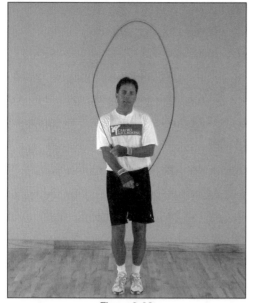

Figure 3-88

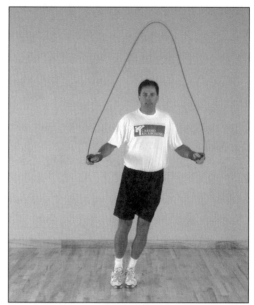

Figure 3-89

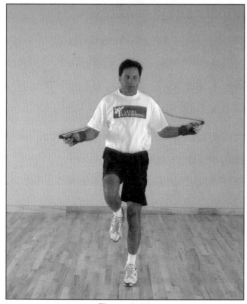

Figure 3-90

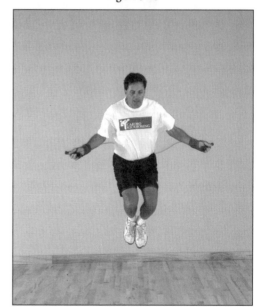

Figure 3-91

HELPFUL HINTS FOR SKIPPING ROPE

There are two important hints to successful and effective rope skipping.

- Learn to get in and out of the rope using the figure-eight, so that when you miss, you do not have to start all over again. See Figures 3-93 and 3-94.

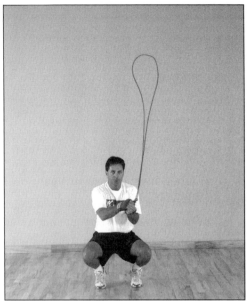

Figure 3-92

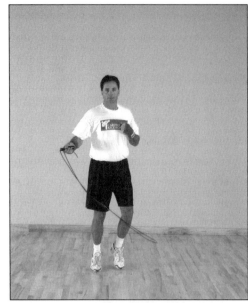

Figure 3-93

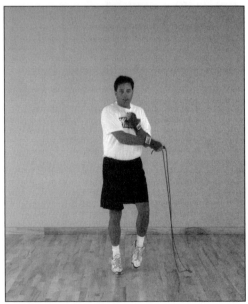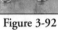

Figure 3-94

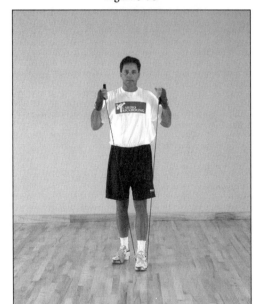

Figure 3-95

- The rope should be sized so that the handles are at least shoulder height when you step into the rope with one foot, Figure 3-95.

MAJOR MUSCLES WORKED IN KICKBOXING

Each fundamental technique exercises particular muscle groups. For your information, they are described below.

1. Punches

Jab. Your shoulder flexes, beginning the movement. To do this, your anterior deltoid and medial deltoid are innervated. Your triceps brachii extend your elbow to complete your jab.

Cross. Your spine rotates when your internal and external obliques contract to begin your body motion. Then, just as in your jab, contract your anterior and medial deltoids. Finally, your triceps brachii complete the cross.

Hook. Your internal and external obliques begin the movement in your upper body. Then your pectoralis major and anterior deltoid contract simultaneously. Your serratus, anterior, and medial deltoid remain contracted as you complete the hook.

Uppercut. Your internal and external obliques begin the movement in your upper body. Then your medial and anterior deltoid contract as your elbow remains flexed to complete your uppercut.

2. Kicks

Front kick. Your iliopsoas (hip flexor) and rectus femoris raise your knee into a fold position. Then your quadriceps contract to extend your knee. Your hamstrings stop your contraction and actually help pull your extended foot back into a flexed knee position. Finally, your iliopsoas and rectus femoris contract to return your foot to its original position.

Roundhouse. Your first movement is hip abduction. This concentric contraction involves your gluteus medius and tensor fasciae latae. Simultaneously, your iliopsoas and rectus femoris contract. Just as in your front kick, your quadriceps are responsible for knee extension. At the completion of your kick, your hamstrings are also involved in retracting your foot back into your fold position. At the same time, your hip adducts eccentrically and your iliopsoas and rectus femoris also eccentrically contract to return your foot to its original position.

Sidekick. Your sidekick begins by concentrically contracting your iliopsoas (hip flexor) and rectus femoris to bring your foot to the fold position. Then, your tensor fasciae latae and gluteus medius are responsible for abducting your hip. Your quadriceps extend your knee to complete your sidekick. Then your gluteus medius and tensor fasciae latae eccentrically contract to adduct your hip. And at the same time, your quadriceps return your foot to its original position by extending your knee back to the floor.

CHAPTER 4

General Description of the Workout

Now that you have covered the basics, you need a general understanding of the flow of a class. You need to know what to expect and to understand why you are doing it.

CLASSES

In my program, the classes last one hour each—and the instructors and students strictly adhere to this timeframe. Additionally, the protocol for *Cardio Kickboxing®* classes in a health club versus learning kickboxing in a martial arts school or gym is different. These differences are described below.

1. You often learn the basics by imitating your instructor who will have little time for detailed explanation or application of the techniques you are learning during the warm up and review component of the class.

2. The class format will include the following phases:
   - warm-up
   - review
   - workout
   - conditioning and strengthening
   - tapering and cool-down

3. *Cardio Kickboxing®* classes are much less formal than martial arts classes. There are no belts awarded, and no uniforms are worn. Whatever you normally wear to work out is acceptable.

4. Athletic shoes (especially cross trainers that do not have as much tread as running shoes) are a must for these classes, particularly when skipping rope or kicking the bags.

5. Music is a great tool for motivating you to work a little harder. It also adds excitement to the class.

PREPARATION

For sanitary and safety purposes, purchase a pair of your own personal hand-wraps and quality training gloves. See Appendix for some recommendations. Also purchase a jump rope. PVC speed ropes can easily be adjusted to your own height.

Prior to the class, wrap both of your hands with cloth handwraps to help protect the knuckles and support the wrists. Keep your bag gloves and jump rope in close proximity to you to avoid delays when moving from one segment of the workout to the other.

WARM-UP

Classes begin with a three to five minute warm-up and then go directly into drills that loosen you up and synchronize movement for the upper and lower body. During the warm-up, emphasis is first placed on sliding your feet and pivoting while avoiding crossing your feet. Then, bobbing and weaving sequences are done. Instead of using traditional stretch kicks used in most martial arts classes, the class includes much safer knee-ups. Knee-ups are done by bringing the knee into the chest to stretch the hamstrings and glutes.

REVIEW

A review of the five basic punches (jab, cross, hook, uppercut, and spinning backfist) is performed. The class follows the instructor who covers a variety of punching combinations. You should then expect to review the front kick, round-house, and lead-leg sidekick. So that the workout becomes kickboxing as opposed to boxing or karate, a series of basic hand-and-foot combinations are completed such as a left front kick/jab/cross punch or jab/cross punch/right roundhouse kick. These basic sequences should feel natural with the punches and kicks flowing one after the other.

Beginners should be cautious when punching or kicking in the air, as opposed to making contact with a target. Do not fully extend your arms or legs when throwing punches and kicks. Full extension of the arm when punching or leg while kicking could cause hyperextension of an elbow or knee. Shadowboxing and shadow kickboxing with an emphasis on foot movement, particularly side-to-side and in-and-out movements, enable you to blend all the techniques into a polished intense cardiovascular routine.

WORKOUT PHASE

Circuit training and bag work. The circuit training format with all the variable stations allows individuals to work at their own skill and fitness level. If you are in great shape, you can work harder; if you are just getting started, you can work less vigorously and focus on polishing your punches and kicks. You will usually be working at two-minute intervals (rounds). If you are not used to punching and kicking a bag, these two minutes can be the longest two minutes of your life. Gradually, however, your body will get used to this new sensation.

Each bag also has a different function. Some develop power; others are for hand/eye coordination, and others improve punching and kicking accuracy. After you are comfortable with doing the *Cardio Kickboxing®* circuit, try not to sustain a flat linear pace. Instead, add bursts of intensity within the round itself to simulate real life action in the ring or in the event of an attack by incorporating speed-punch and power-punch drills during your rounds.

The one-on-one station with the instructor using punch mitts or kicking pad puts all the techniques into perspective with the focus on movement and distance. This is where you learn balance and distance and where you simulate real life action as the instructor constantly moves and makes technical corrections. You receive positive reinforcement and feedback to correct your technique each time, which quickly improves your skill and confidence level. For the more seasoned participants, your instructor may even put on some protective gear.

This modified sparring component—trying to punch or kick a moving person—takes you to a higher level. Most people are surprised at how difficult it is to land their techniques effectively on a moving target. At the same time, your instructor may throw some punches and kicks in your direction (without making contact) so that while you are attacking, you do not attack with impunity. Instead, you have to calculate when to attack and when to defend. Frankly, this one-on-one attention combined with the ability to workout at your own pace makes this a unique approach to participating in a group fitness class.

Actual sparring is not a requirement of the class since most of the members are not competitive kickboxers, and, in fact, are active members of the workforce. You certainly are not about to go to work the next day with abrasions on your face, a puffy nose, or sore feet (from kicking barefoot while sparring as in a traditional martial arts class). In fact, the more protection and padding for the hands and feet, the better.

CONDITIONING AND STRENGTHENING

After the circuit training on the various stations, you will come back together as a group to do some additional conditioning drills, plyometric exercises, or skipping rope. Push-ups and/or crunches may also be added.

TAPERING AND COOL-DOWN

To finish the workout, a conventional cool-down period with some upper body, leg, and lower back stretches are incorporated. The intent is to bring your heart rate down to 100 beats per minute or less.

Classes seem to fly by with no time to reflect on work or any other problems that may be causing stress. Once you take five to eight classes, you will begin to feel quite comfortable with the routine. You may even begin to notice some minor physical changes. Your instructor will add variety to the class to keep it fresh. The classes will generally follow this format. However, each class may vary somewhat to include more drills or new techniques referred to as *add-ons* as discussed in Chapters 6 and 7.

ATTITUDE

There are 110-pound, experienced women practitioners that can punch harder than 180-pound novice men; the difference is technique. There are also 50-year-old, 200-pound men in these classes that are in better shape than many of their 25-year-old counterparts; the difference here is attitude. As experts in the industry know, fitness does not occur overnight, particularly if there has been a long sedentary period before an adult gets back on the exercise wagon. If you go by the motto that conditioning is the S-L-O-W adaptation of your body to (physical) stress, you will enjoy these classes much more and soon reap the benefits of *Cardio Kickboxing*®.

CHAPTER 5

Basic Workout Outline

BASIC WORKOUT FORMAT

A. Warm-up: 8 minutes

    Step 1. Warm-up routine

    Step 2. Punching drills

    Step 3. Stance and foot movement

    Step 4. Bobbing and weaving

B. Review: 12 minutes

    Step 5. Five basic punches

    Step 6. Punching combinations

    Step 7. Shadow boxing

    Step 8. Knee-ups

    Step 9. Three basic kicks

    Step 10. Punching and kicking combinations

C. Workout: 25 minutes

    Step 11. Shadow kickboxing

    Step 12. Circuit training/ bag work

D. Conditioning and Strengthening: 10 minutes

    Step 13. Speed punching drills; power punching drills

    Step 14. Speed kicking drills; power kicking drills

    Step 15. Skipping rope

    Step 16. Plyometric exercises

    Step 17. Crunches and pushups

E. Tapering and Cool-Down Phase: 5 minutes

    Step 18. Upper body stretches

    Step 19. Torso and lower body stretches

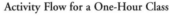

Activity Flow for a One-Hour Class

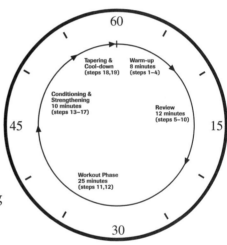

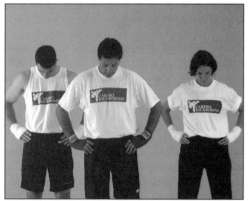

Figure 5-1a

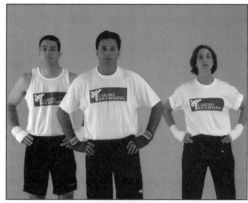

Figure 5-1b

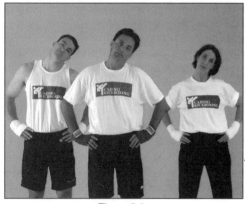

Figure 5-2a

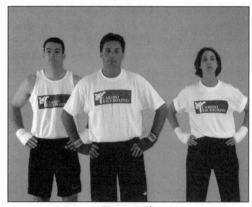

Figure 5-2b

WARM-UP (STEPS 1-4)

Step 1. Warm-up routine. This routine should also be used at the end of the workout. We use it here to allow those who are late for class or who are still wrapping their hands more time to get ready.

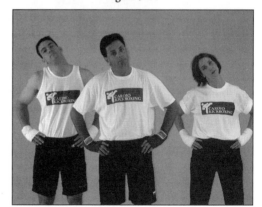

Figure 5-2c

a. Tilt your head forward and back 4 times. See Figure 5-1a, b Tilt your head left to center, right to center 4 times. See Figure 5-2a, b, c. Turn your head left to center and right to center 4 times. See Figure 5-3a, b, c. Finally, Rotate left to right and right to left 4 times. See Figure 5-4a, b.

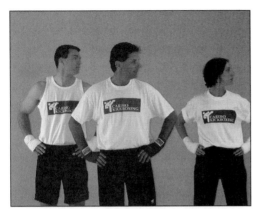

Figure 5-3a

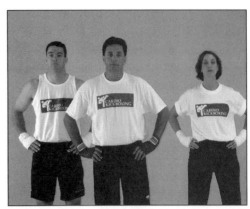

Figure 5-3b

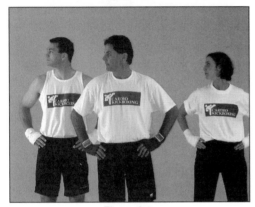

Figure 5-3c

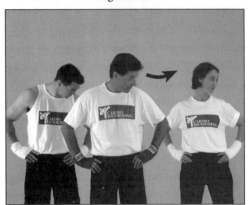

Figure 5-4a

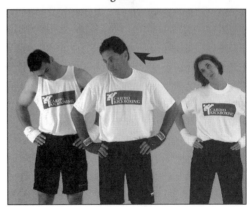

Figure 5-4b

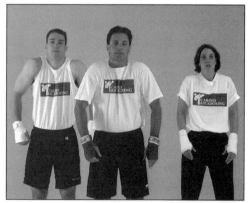

Figure 5-5a

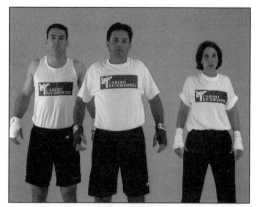

Figure 5-5b

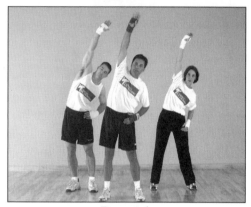

Figure 5-6a

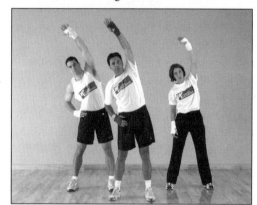

Figure 5-6b

b. Rotate shoulders forward and backward 4 times each. See Figure 5-5a, b.

c. Stretch up with your right arm and pulse 4 times and then stretch up with your left arm and pulse four times. See Figure 5-6a, b.

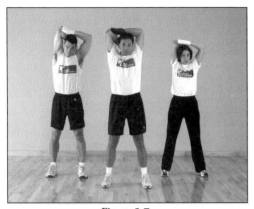

Figure 5-7a

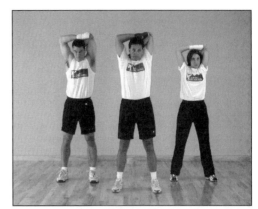

Figure 5-7b

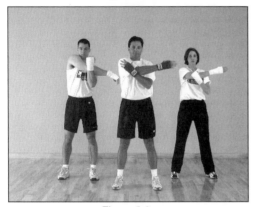

Figure 5-8a

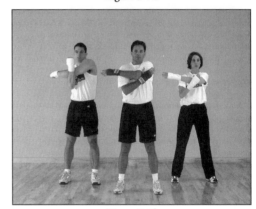

Figure 5-8b

d. Stretch your right tricep and then stretch your left tricep. Hold each for 10 seconds. See Figure 5-7a, b.

e. Stretch your right arm horizontally, and then stretch your left arm horizontally. Hold each for 10 seconds. See Figure 5-8a, b.

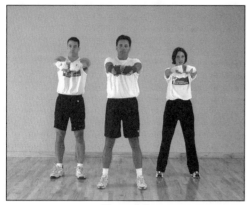

Figure 5-9

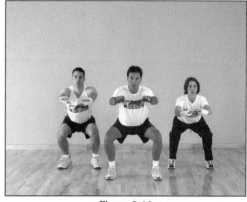

Figure 5-10

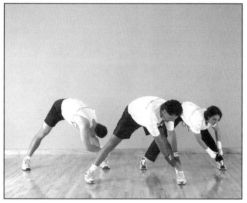

Figure 5-11a

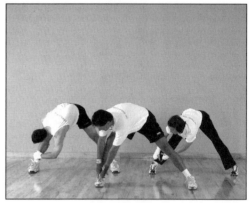

Figure 5-11b

f. Lock your fingers for a forward press. See Figure 5-9.

g. Squats 8 times. See Figure 5-10.

h. Hamstring stretch (see Figure 5-11a, b) and 4 hip flexor pushes (see Figure 5-12).

i. Full circular trunk rotation left to right (4 times) and right to left (4 times). See Figure 5-13.

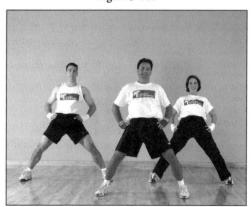

Figure 5-12

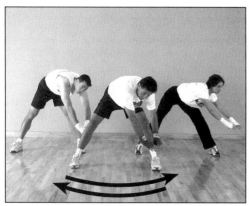

Figure 5-13

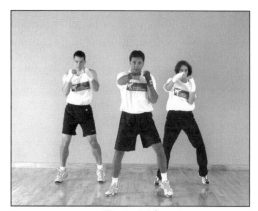

Figure 5-14

Step 2. Punching Drills. These are not authentic punches, but drills to warm up only. Punch lightly, synchronizing your foot movement with the timing of your punching.

a. Straight punch drill. Start with your feet parallel shoulder width apart. Punch regular speed and rapid-fire straight-line punches parallel to the floor. Perform these in place keeping the opposite hand next to the face (24-32

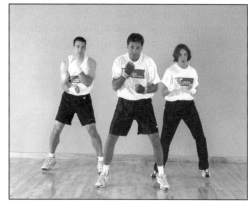

Figure 5-15

times). See Figure 5-14. Be sure to rotate your fists so that they finish with the palms down. Keep your elbows in, chin down, and back slightly bent. Move forward and back 4 times, and left and right 4 times while continuously punching.

b. Uppercut drill. Place feet parallel and shoulder-width apart; punch perpendicular to the floor with palms facing the body, elbows in, chin down, back slightly bent. Punch regular speed 24-32 times and rapid-fire 16 times. Perform each set three times. See Figure 5-15.

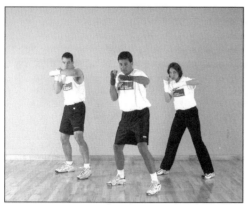

Figure 5-16a

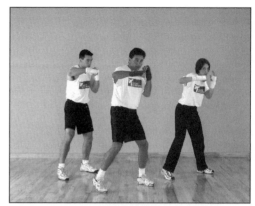

Figure 5-16b

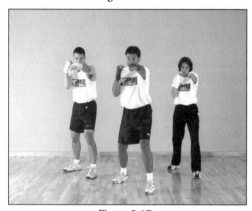

Figure 5-17a

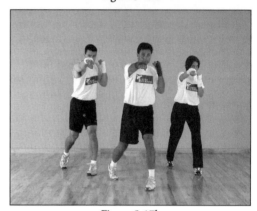

Figure 5-17b

c. Hooking drill. Assume normal stance, and step at 45° angle; pivot and hook. Use the hips for power, and keep your arm parallel to the floor, palm down. Your non-punching hand stays up next to the cheek. Alternate left and right, and perform each 8 times. See Figures 5-16a, b.

d. Hip rotation drill side to side. Assume normal stance, and jab-cross. Pivot to the right on the balls of your feet. Punch left, rotate, pivot, and punch right. Look in the direction of the punch and exaggerate your hip movements. Perform 8 sets. See Figures 5-17a, b, c, d.

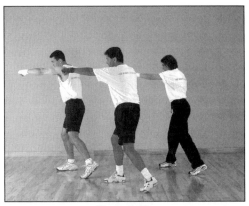

Figure 5-17c

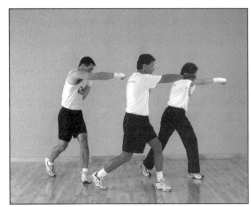

Figure 5-17d

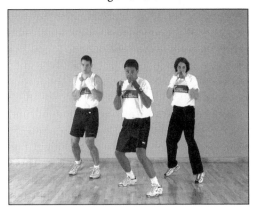

Figure 5-18

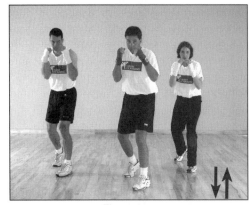

Figure 5-19

Step 3. Stance and Foot Movement.

a. Bouncing in place. Assume normal stance, and bounce 8 times in place to warm up the calves. See Figure 5-18. Move up and bounce 8 more times. Switch sides, and bounce in place 8 times, and then move up and bounce 8 more times. Repeat for 2 sets on each side.

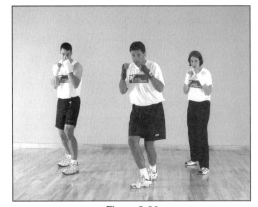

Figure 5-20

b. Slide. Assume normal stance, and slide forward and backward 4 times. See Figure 5-19. Do not cross your feet. See Figure 5-20.

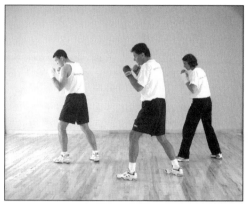

Figure 5-21

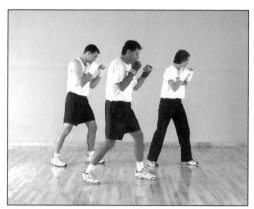

Figure 5-22

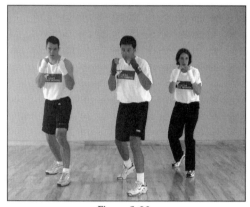

Figure 5-23a

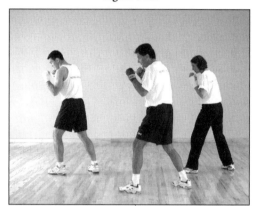

Figure 5-23b

c. Pivoting.

- Slide forward, and pivot clockwise left 90° off the lead left foot. See Figure 5-21. Return and slide back. Repeat for 3 sets.

- Slide forward, pivot counterclockwise right 90° off the left lead foot. See Figure 5-22. Return and slide back. Repeat for 3 sets.

- Combine the slides forward and backward with left and right pivot. Perform 3 sets. See Figure 5-23a, b, c, d.

d. Lateral movement

- Circle left, and then circle right, pushing off the opposite foot (6 times). See Figure 5-24a, b.

- Combine lateral movement with sliding in and out (6 times). Optional.

Step 4. Bobbing and Weaving. From your neutral stance, bend at your knees and lower back. Perform the exercises first individually and then together as a sequence.

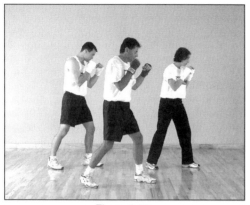

Figure 5-23c

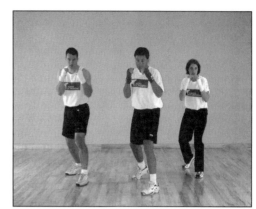

Figure 5-23d

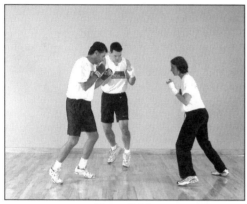

Figure 5-24a

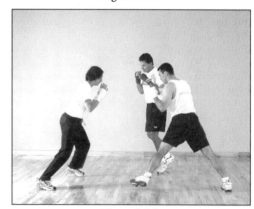

Figure 5-24b

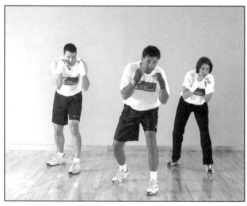

Figure 5-25a

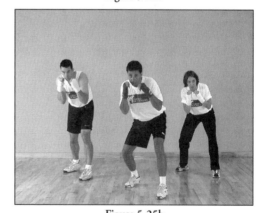

Figure 5-25b

a. Left at a 45° angle (4 times). See Figure 5-25a.

b. Right at a 45° angle (4 times). See Figure 5-25b.

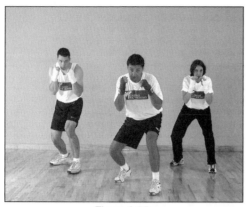

Figure 5-25c

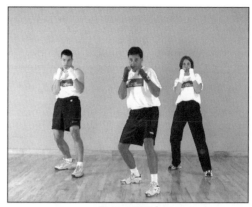

Figure 5-25d

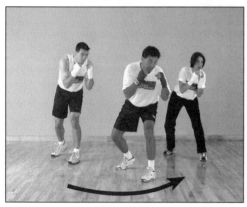

Figure 5-25e

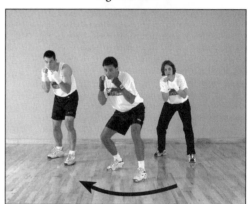

Figure 5-25f

c. Straight down (4 times). See Figure 5-25c.

d. Lean back (4 times). See Figure 5-25d.

e. Weave left (4 times). See Figure 5-25e.

f. Weave right (4 times). See Figure 5-25f.

g. Sequence steps (a) through (f) and perform each sequence 8 times.

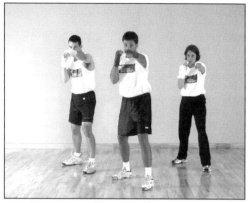

Figure 5-26a

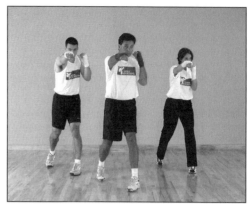

Figure 5-26b

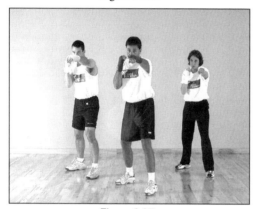

Figure 5-27a

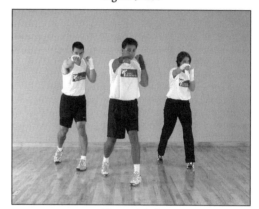

Figure 5-27b

REVIEW (STEPS 5-10)

Step 5. Five Basic Punches. Perform each of the five basic punches 8 times each (4 times for the spinning backfist). Start first with the jab, then continue with the cross, hook, uppercut, and spinning backfist. Except for the spinning backfist (because you will get dizzy), you can increase the repetitions from an 8 count for beginners to a 16 or 24 count as you become more fit.

Step 6. Punching Combinations

a. Jab/cross (8 times). See Figures 5-26a, b.

b. Jab/cross/hook (8 times). See Figures 5-27a, b, c.

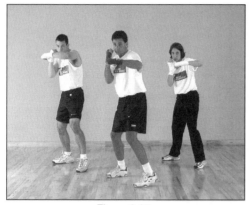

Figure 5-27c

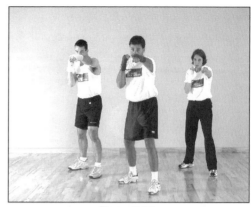

Figure 5-28a

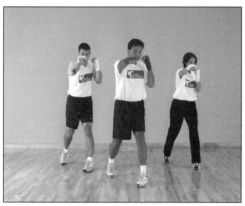

Figure 5-28b

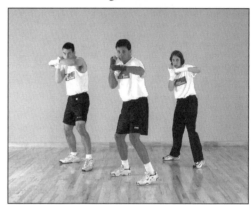

Figure 5-28c

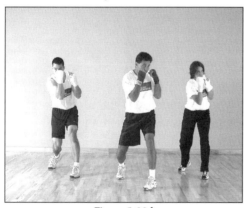

Figure 5-28d

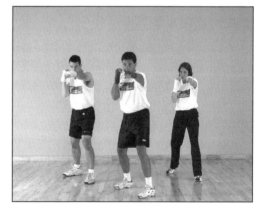

Figure 5-29

c. Jab/cross/hook/uppercut (8 times). See Figures 5-28a, b, c, d.

d. Double jab (8 times). See Figure 5-29.

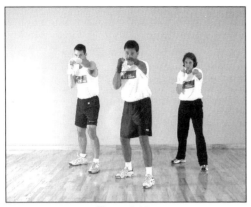

Figure 5-30a

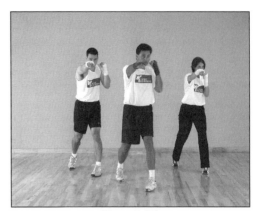

Figure 5-30b

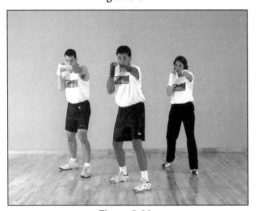

Figure 5-30c

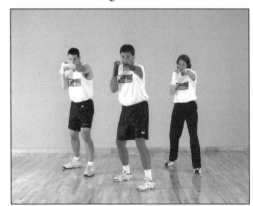

Figure 5-31a

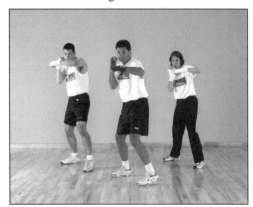

Figure 5-31b

e. Jab/cross/jab (8 times). See Figures 5-30a, b, c.

f. Jab/left hook (8 times). See Figures 5-31a, b.

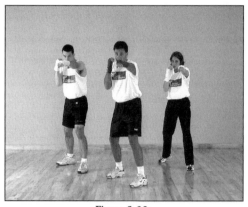

Figure 5-32a

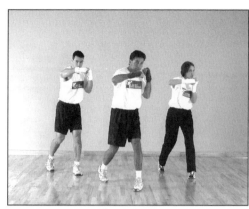

Figure 5-32b

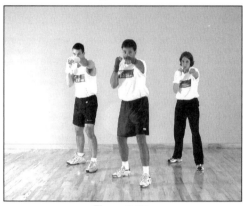

Figure 5-33a

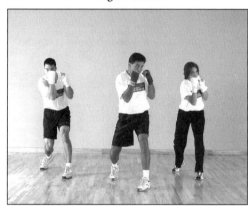

Figure 5-33b

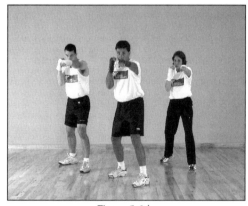

Figure 5-34a

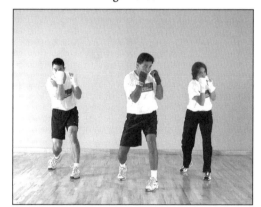

Figure 5-34b

g. Jab/right hook (8 times). See Figures 5-32a, b.

h. Jab/right uppercut (8 times). See Figures 5-33a, b.

i. Jab/right uppercut—left hook (8 times). See Figures 5-34a, b, c.

j. Right uppercut/left uppercut (8 times). See Figures 5-35a, b.

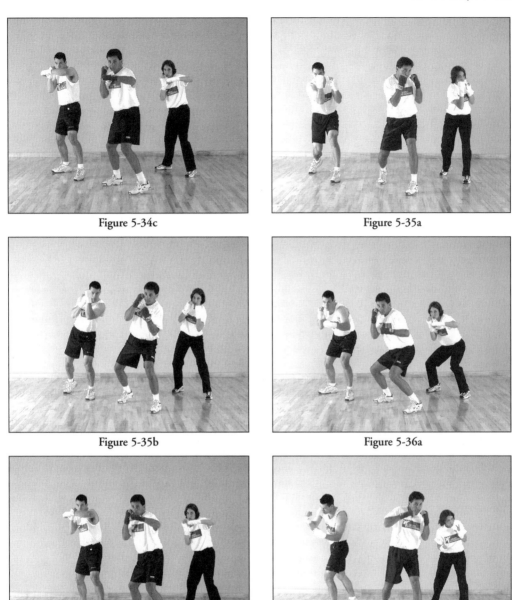

Figure 5-34c

Figure 5-35a

Figure 5-35b

Figure 5-36a

Figure 5-36b

Figure 5-37

k. Double left hook—body, head (8 times). See Figures 5-36a, b.

Step 7. Shadow boxing, 1-3 rounds. Combine foot movement, bobbing and weaving, and punching combinations. See Figure 5-37.

75

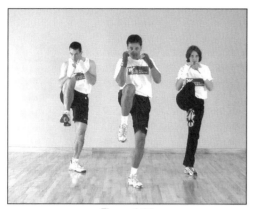

Figure 5-38

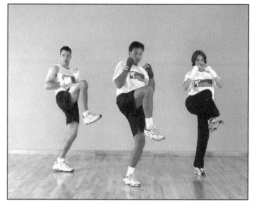

Figure 5-39a

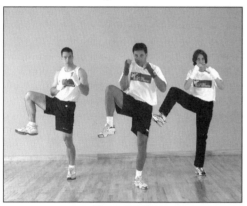

Figure 5-39b

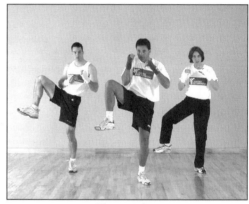

Figure 5-40a

Step 8. Knee-ups. Knee-ups warm-up and stretch primarily your hamstrings. This exercise also trains you to initiate the front kick by bringing up the knee (similar to bouncing a soccer ball off the knee).

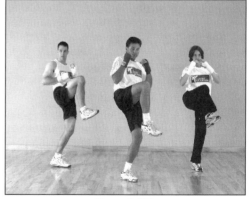

Figure 5-40b

a. Bring the knee straight up into the chest, 8 times each knee. See Figure 5-38.

b. Circle the knee toward the center of the body and out, 8 times each knee. See Figure 5-39a, b.

c. Circle the knee away from the body and toward the center, 8 times each knee. See Figure 5-40a, b.

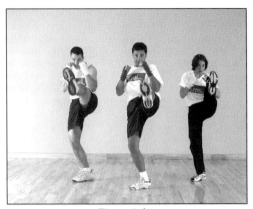

Figure 5-41a

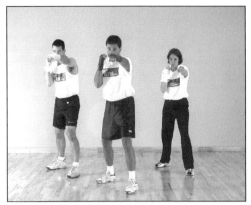

Figure 5-41b

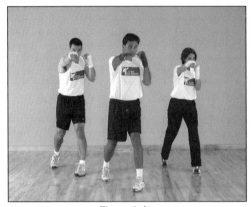

Figure 5-41c

Step 9. Three Basic Kicks

a. Lead-leg front kick, then rear-leg front kick, (8 times each leg).

b. Lead-leg roundhouse kick, then rear-leg roundhouse kick (8 times each leg).

c. Lead-leg sidekick (8 times).

Step 10. Punching and Kicking Combinations.

a. Left front kick/jab/cross (8 times). See Figures 5-41a, b, c.

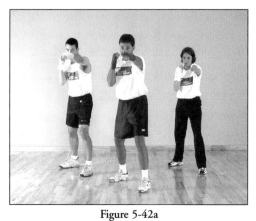

Figure 5-42a

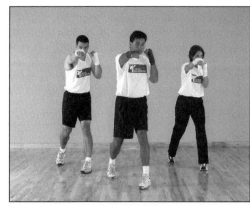

Figure 5-42b

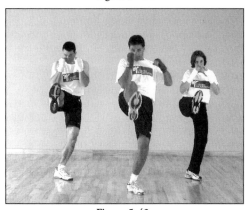

Figure 5-42c

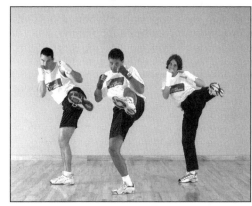

Figure 5-43a

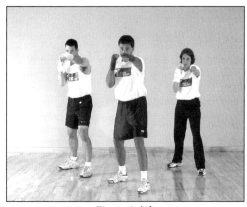

Figure 5-43b

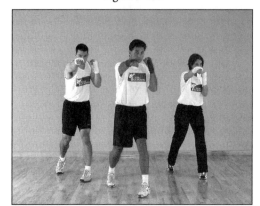

Figure 5-43c

b. Jab/cross/right front kick (8 times). See Figures 5-42a, b, c.

c. Left roundhouse kick/jab/cross (8 times). See Figures 5-43a, b, c.

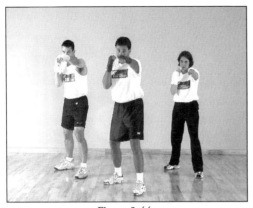

Figure 5-44a

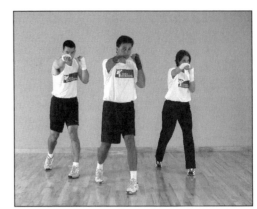

Figure 5-44b

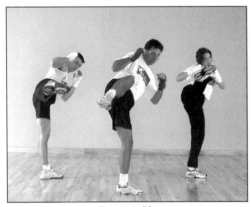

Figure 5-44c

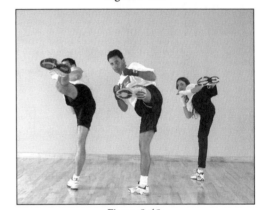

Figure 5-45a

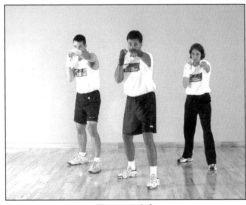

Figure 5-45b

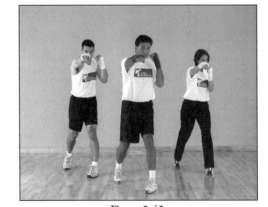

Figure 5-45c

d. Jab/cross/right roundhouse kick (8 times). See Figures 5-44a, b, c.

e. Lead-leg/sidekick/jab/cross (8 times). See Figures 5-45a, b, c.

WORKOUT (STEPS 11-12)

Step 11. Shadow kickboxing (1–3 rounds). Combine foot movement, bobbing and weaving, punching and kicking combinations.

Step 12. Circuit training (8–10 rounds). Normally, this program uses a sequence of two-minute rounds with a 30-second break. The number of stations, equipment and participants will vary among sites so that adjustments will be made. Push-ups, crunches, and standing stretches can be done between rounds (instead of the rest period) or at the end of the class. (The rest period would need to be extended from 30 seconds to 45 or 60 if they're being done between rounds.) See Figure 5-46.

CONDITIONING AND STRENGTHENING (STEPS 13-17)

Step 13. Punching

a. Speed-punching drill (30 seconds; 4 times). These are rapid-fire punches thrown in bunches in the air, but normally on the heavybag or punch mitts.

b. Power-punching drill (8–12 punches; 4 times). These are hard punches thrown flat footed for more power on the heavybag.

Step 14. Kicking

a. Speed-kicking drill (8–12 rapid-fire front kicks, 3 times left; 3 times right).

b. Power-kicking drill (8–12 power front kicks, 3 times left; 3 times right).

Step 15. Skipping rope. Use a figure-eight to get comfortable with the rope; to rest; or to keep the rhythm if you miss. (Perform 1–3 two- or three-minute rounds).

Step 16. Plyometric and leg-strengthening exercises. These exercises can be done with your hands behind your head, on your hips or in the on-guard position. Plyometric and leg-strengthening exercises were designed to help develop explosiveness and power when kicking.

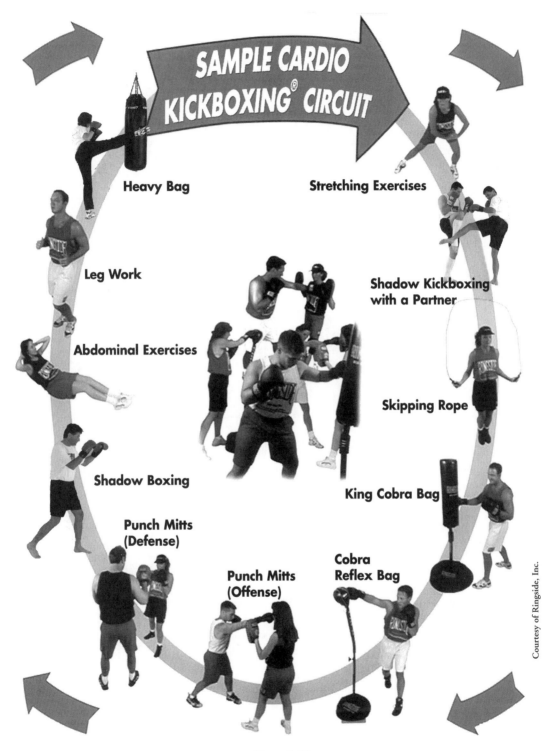

SAMPLE CARDIO KICKBOXING® CIRCUIT

Heavy Bag

Stretching Exercises

Leg Work

Shadow Kickboxing with a Partner

Abdominal Exercises

Skipping Rope

Shadow Boxing

King Cobra Bag

Punch Mitts (Defense)

Punch Mitts (Offense)

Cobra Reflex Bag

Courtesy of Ringside, Inc.

Figure 5-46

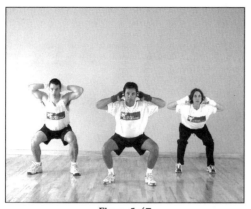

Figure 5-47

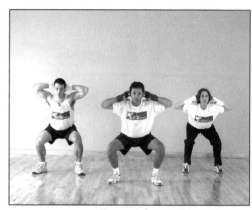

Figure 5-48a

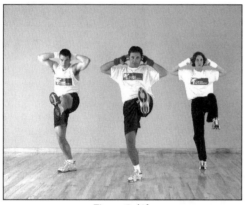

Figure 5-48b

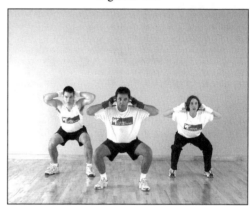

Figure 5-49a

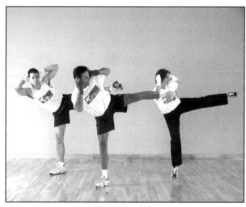

Figure 5-49b

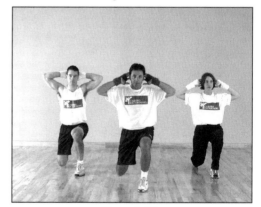

Figure 5-50a

a. Squats (8 times). See Figure 5-47.

b. Squats with front kick, (8 times left, 8 times right). See Figures 5-48a, b.

c. Squats with sidekick, (8 times left, 8 times right). See Figures 5-49a, b.

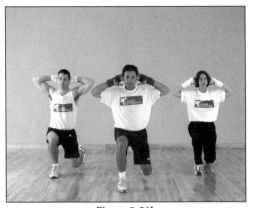

Figure 5-50b

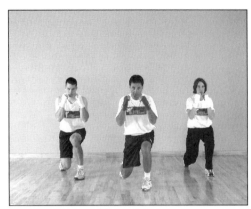

Figure 5-51a

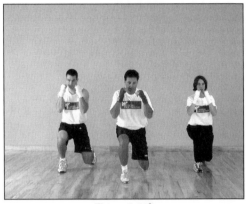

Figure 5-51b

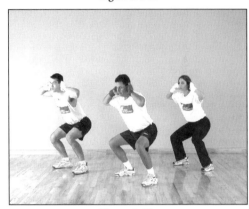

Figure 5-52a

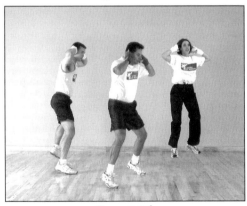

Figure 5-52b

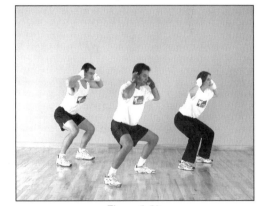

Figure 5-52c

d. Alternating lunges (8 times left, 8 times right). See Figure 5-50a, b.

e. Knee dips (8 times left, 8 times right). See Figure 5-51a, b.

f. Jump and switch (8 times corner to corner). See Figures 5-52a, b, c.

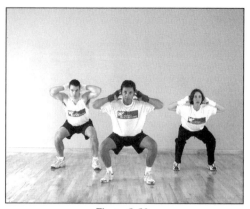

Figure 5-53a

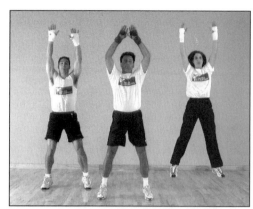

Figure 5-53b

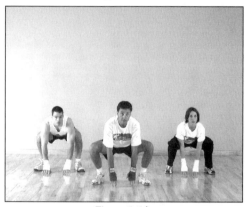

Figure 5-54a

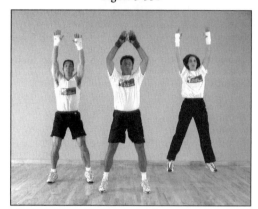

Figure 5-54b

g. Squat, straight up jump (8 times). See Figure 5-53a, b.

h. Squat, tap the floor and jump (8 times). See Figures 5-54a, b.

Step 17. Crunches and Push-ups (Caution: Heart rate check, do not begin until your heart rate is below 100).

a. Various sets of crunches; strive for quality, not quantity, contracting your abs with little head and neck effort (use a mat when performing crunches at the end of the class, not when doing them between rounds).

- Pulse up with your arms passing between your knees (25 times). See Figure 5-55a.

- Cross your arms over your chest (25 times). See Figure 5-55b.

- Put your ankle on your opposite knee; fingertips behind your ears and twist up to work your external obliques (15 times each side). See Figure 5-55c.

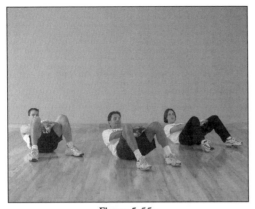

Figure 5-55a

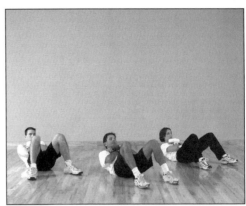

Figure 5-55b

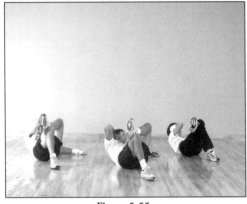

Figure 5-55c

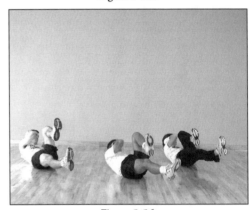

Figure 5-56a

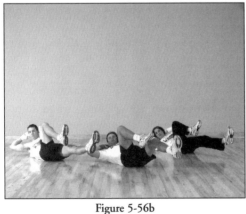

Figure 5-56b

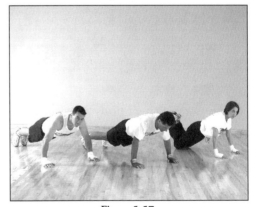

Figure 5-57a

- Bicycles (one set of 100, single count). See Figure 5-56a, b.

b. Regular or modified push-ups (3 sets as follows: 15 times, then 10 times, then 5 times). See Figures 5-57a, b.

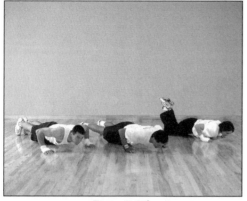

Figure 5-57b

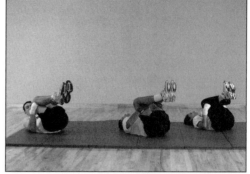

Figure 5-58a

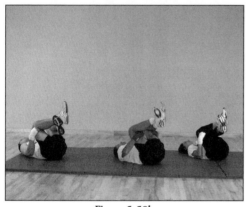

Figure 5-58b

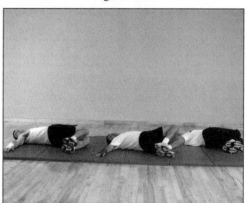

Figure 5-59a

TAPERING AND COOL-DOWN (STEP 18)

Step 18. Upper body stretches. These stretches can also be modified and done from a sitting position.

Repeat Step 1, Warm-up. See Figures 5-1 through 5-13.

Step 19. Lower body stretches. Hold each stretch for 10–20 seconds.

a. Bring the knees straight back into the chest and/or with legs crossed. See Figure 5-58a, b.

b. Drop the knees left and right keeping the shoulder blades on the floor. See Figure 5-59a, b.

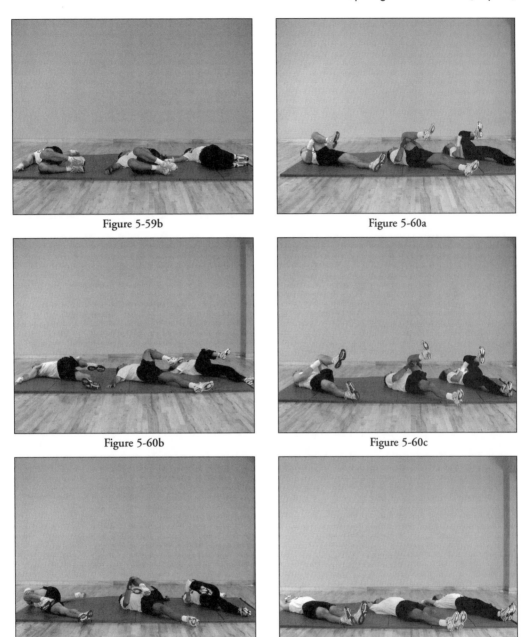

Figure 5-59b

Figure 5-60a

Figure 5-60b

Figure 5-60c

Figure 5-60d

Figure 5-61

c. Bring the knee into chest; knee across the chest. See Figure 5-60a, b, c, d.

d. Full stretch. See Figure 5-61.

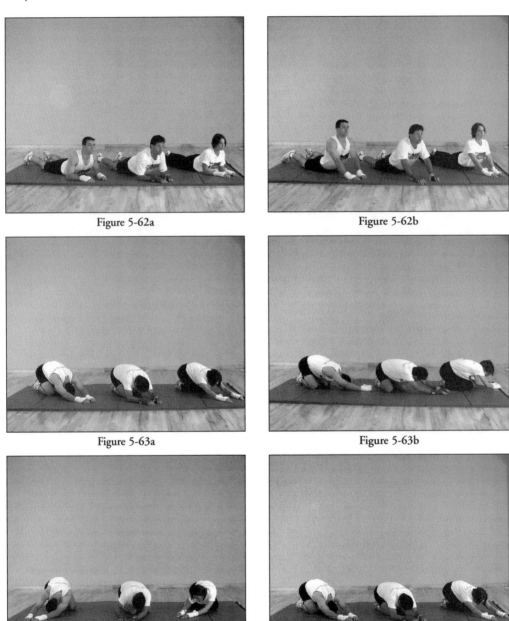

Figure 5-62a

Figure 5-62b

Figure 5-63a

Figure 5-63b

Figure 5-63c

Figure 5-63d

e. Roll over to stomach. Perform back hyperextension stretch. See Figures 5-62a, b.

f. Slide up and tuck knees to stretch the lower back: center, left, right, center. See Figures 5-63a, b, c, d.

CHAPTER 6

Intermediate Techniques

The following "add-ons" can be added to or substituted in the basic workout format.

They are not difficult techniques or concepts to learn. Some require working with a partner, and some can be done individually in a class setting. *For your reference, the step number from the original workout described in Chapter 5 is indicated at the beginning of each add-on.*

Step 3. Foot movement. (refer to page 67)

e. Cutting off the ring. Stepping in the direction of an opponent who is circling and using a lot of movement. The application for the sport is to intercept and force the opponent into action (see Figure 6-1a, b). From a fitness point of view, the more you move the better the workout—as with sliding, pivoting, and lateral movement.

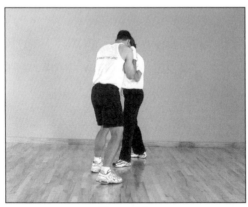

Figure 6-1a

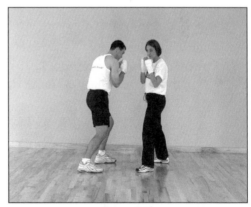

Figure 6-1b

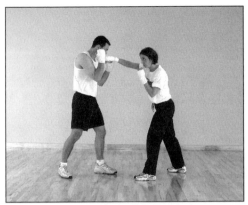
Figure 6-2a

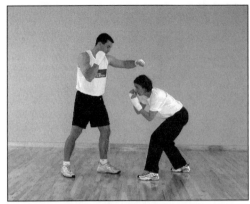
Figure 6-2b

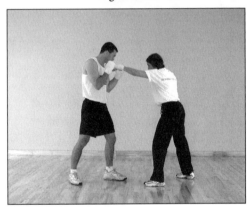
Figure 6-2c

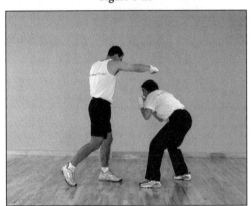
Figure 6-2d

Step 4. Bobbing and weaving. (refer to page 68)

h. Punching and weaving. See Figure 6-2a, b, c, d. Rather than punch and stop, it is better to keep your head moving after you finish a punching combination while still in range to avoid getting hit.

i. Feinting. See Figure 6-3a, b. Feinting is the act of drawing in your opponent by having him or her react to a subtle fake. Your opponent thinks you are doing one thing when you actually intend to do another attacking technique. For example, feint (fake) a jab and immediately throw a cross.

Step 5. Punches. (refer to page 71)

f. Elbows. Punches can be converted to elbow strikes. The only difference is the proximity to the target. For example, executing a right elbow is the same as a right cross punch except that you have to be closer to the target. The point of impact is usually the tip of the elbow, but the forearm can also be used.

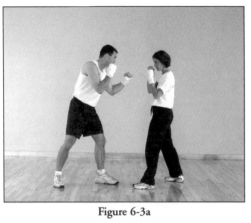

Figure 6-3a

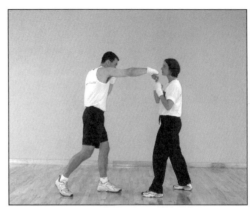

Figure 6-3b

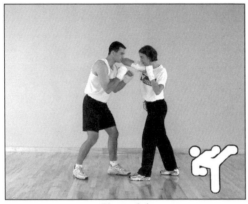

Figure 6-4

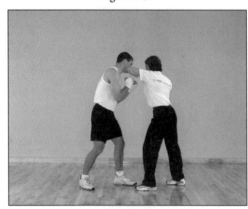

Figure 6-5

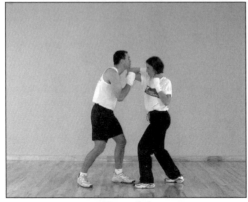

Figure 6-6

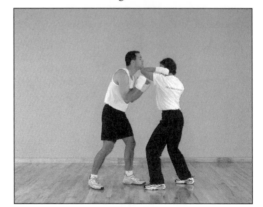

Figure 6-7

- Right elbow. See Figure 6-4.
- Left elbow. See Figure 6-5.
- Right and left rising (uppercut) elbow. See Figures 6-6 and 6-7.

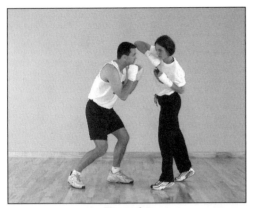

Figure 6-8

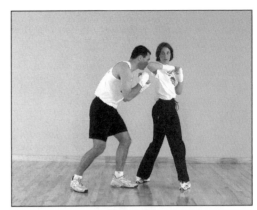

Figure 6-9

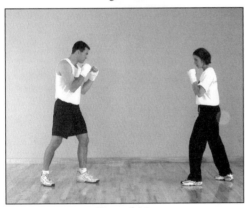

Figure 6-10a

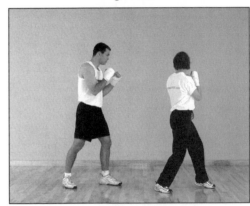

Figure 6-10b

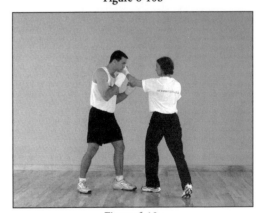

Figure 6-10c

- Chopping elbow. See Figure 6-8.
- Spinning elbow. See Figure 6-9.

g. Step-through Spinning Left Backfist, Attacking. See Figure 6-10a, b, c. Unlike the spinning backfist, which is a counter attack, the step-through backfist is an offensive technique.

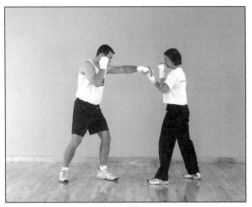

Figure 6-11

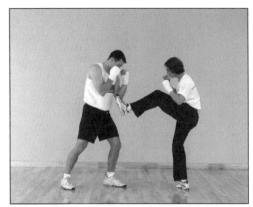

Figure 6-12

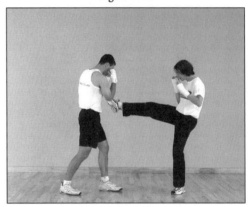

Figure 6-13

h. Parrying. As was mentioned in the fundamentals, parrying is deflecting (not blocking) a punch. See Figure 6-11. The right hand is slightly open and as a jab approaches your chin, your right hand taps it off target. It is often used when you are not quick enough to slip or bob-and-weave away from a punch.

i. Forearm blocking. Also mentioned in the fundamentals, if you cannot move out of range of a kick, you must not drop your hands to block a kick in kickboxing. To do this, you have to parry or actually take the kick on the forearms. To help diminish taking the full effect of the kick on your arms, move slightly away from the kick. This move is similar to rolling with a punch. This may hurt your forearms a bit, but it is safer than having the kick land directly on your ribs or midsection. Absorbing a kick on the forearms will also put you in a position to counter punch effectively.

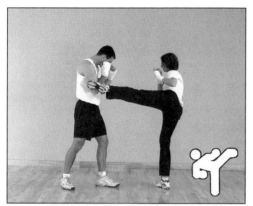

Figure 6-14

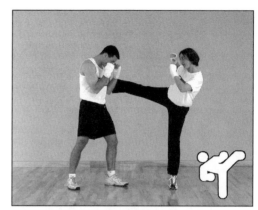

Figure 6-15

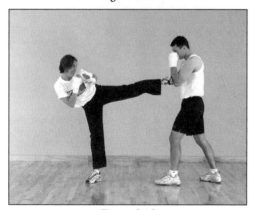

Figure 6-16

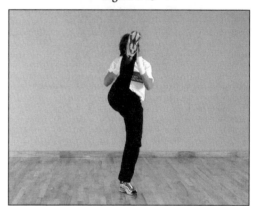

Figure 6-17

- Deflecting a front kick. See Figures 6-12 and 6-13.
- Defending against a roundhouse kick. See Figures 6-14 and 6-15.
- Defending against a sidekick. See Figure 6-16.

Step 8. Stretch kicking. Straight-leg stretch kicking is used to further stretch the hamstrings, but because it is ballistic in nature, it is less safe than the knee-ups. (refer to page 76)

d. Front. See Figure 6-17.

e. In-out. See Figure 6-18.

f. Out-in, Figure 6-19

g. Lateral. See Figure 6-20.

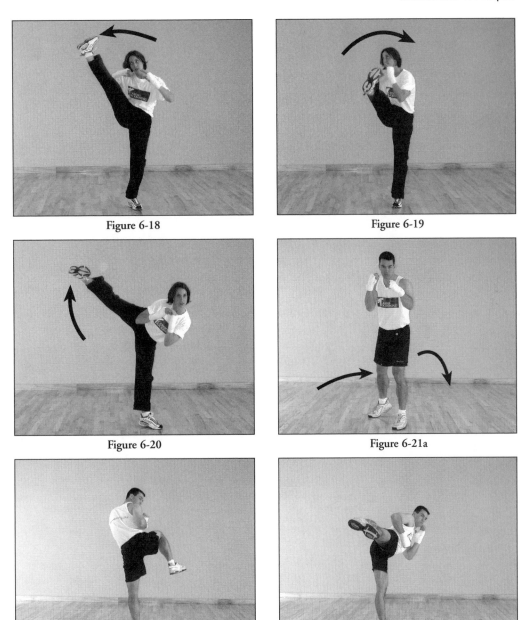

Figure 6-18

Figure 6-19

Figure 6-20

Figure 6-21a

Figure 6-21b

Figure 6-21c

Step 9. Kicks. The spinning sidekick and hook kick are secondary kicks that are thrown infrequently. They are used to give your opponent a different look and may surprise your opponent when they land. Practicing the hook kick helps improve flexibility. (refer to page 77)

d. Spinning sidekick. See Figure 6-21a, b, c.

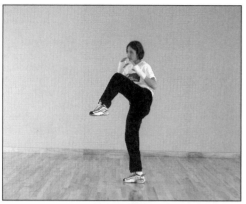

Figure 6-22a

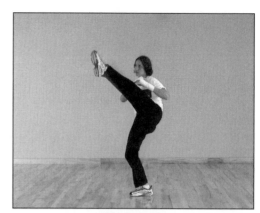

Figure 6-22b

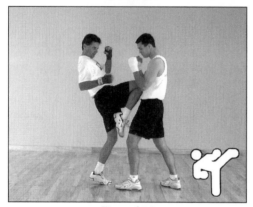

Figure 6-23

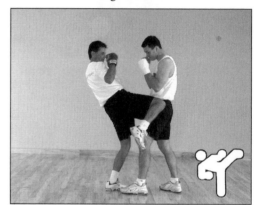

Figure 6-24

e. Hook kick. See Figure 6-22a, b.

f. Knee strikes. Knee strikes are to kicks what elbows are to punches. They can be thrown from the outside or by grabbing your opponent's neck and landing them from the inside.

- Forward. See Figures 6-23.
- 45° angle. See Figure 6-24.

g. Shin blocks. Used to defend against a kick, especially a roundhouse kick, to the legs. See Figure 6-25.

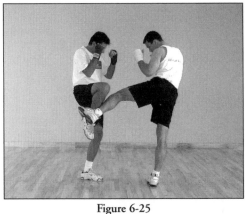

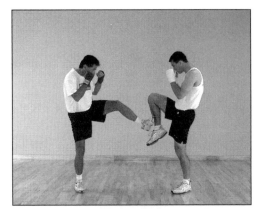

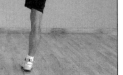

Figure 6-25

Figure 6-26

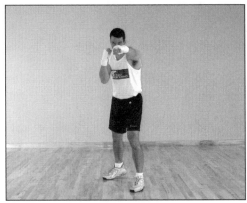

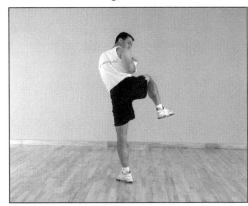

Figure 6-27a

Figure 6-27b

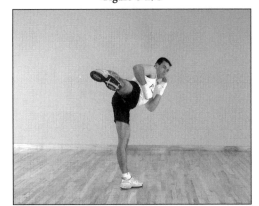

Figure 6-27c

h. Leg checking. Using the bottom of the foot to stop a front kick. It is an illegal technique in the sport of kickboxing, but certainly can be used in a self-defense situation. See Figure 6-26.

Step 10. Punching and kicking combinations. (refer to page 77)

d. Jab/spinning sidekick. See Figures 6-27a, b, c.

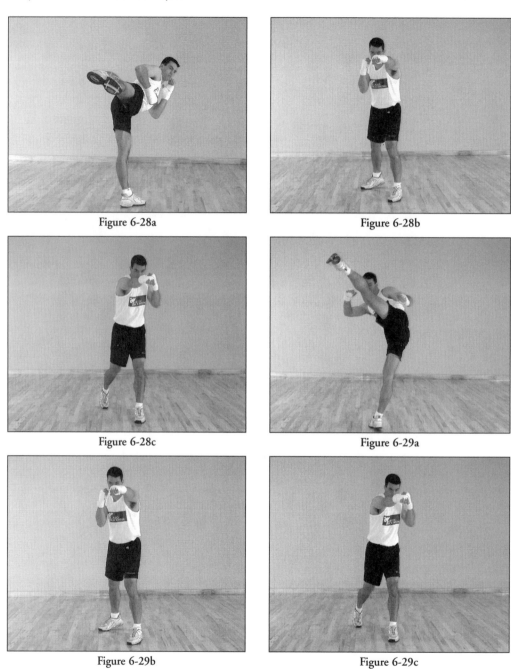

Figure 6-28a

Figure 6-28b

Figure 6-28c

Figure 6-29a

Figure 6-29b

Figure 6-29c

e. Sidekick/spinning sidekick/jab/cross. See Figures 6-28a, b, c.

f. Hook kick/jab/cross. See Figures 6-29a, b, c.

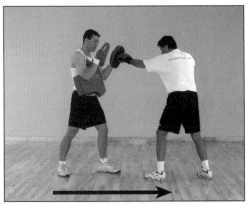

Figure 6-30a

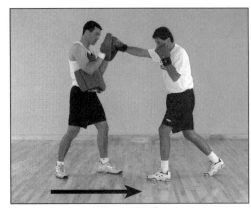

Figure 6-30b

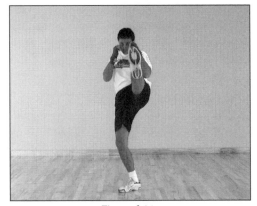

Figure 6-31a

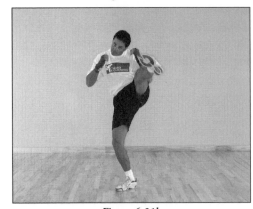

Figure 6-31b

Step 17. Conditioning and Strengthening. These are used as conditioning tools. When you go back to kicking or punching just once, it will be much easier after doing these drills. (refer to page 80)

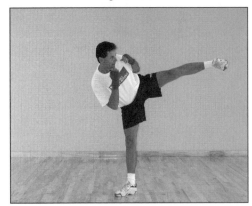

Figure 6-31c

    c. Retreat punching. Strike the punch mitts while moving quickly backward. See Figures 6-30a, b.

    d. Multiple kicking.

      • 10 front, 10 roundhouse, 10 sidekicks in sequence. 3 sets each leg. See Figures 6-31a, b, c.

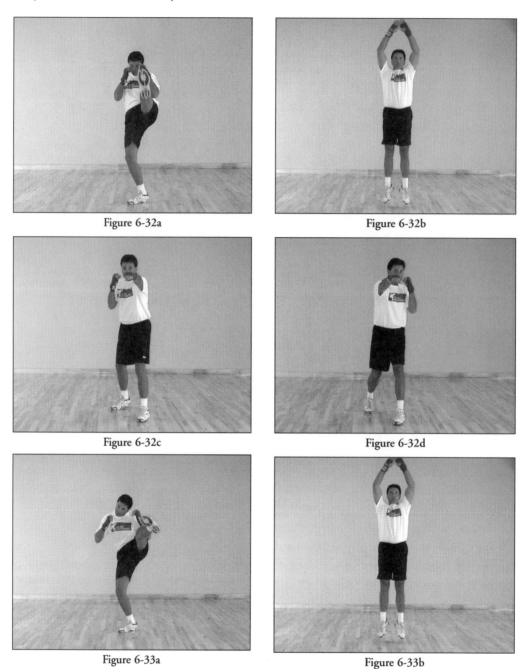

Figure 6-32a

Figure 6-32b

Figure 6-32c

Figure 6-32d

Figure 6-33a

Figure 6-33b

- 5 front kicks, 5 jumps, and 10 straight punches. 3 sets each leg. See Figures 6-32a, b, c, d.

- 5 roundhouse kicks, 5 jumps, and 10 straight punches. See Figures 6-33a, b, c, d.

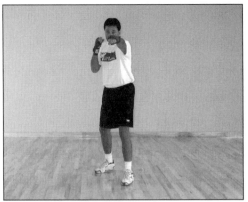

Figure 6-33c

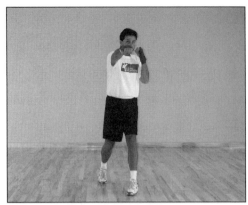

Figure 6-33d

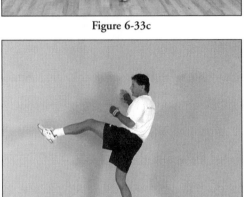

Figure 6-34

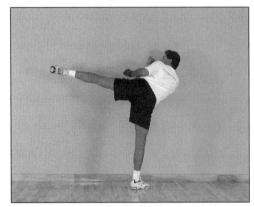

Figure 6-35

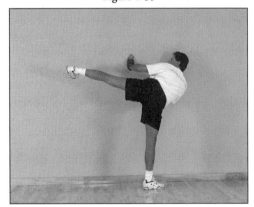

Figure 6-36

e. Slow motion kicking. Great tool for sensing the muscle groups that are used in each individual kick. Plus, kicking slowly improves your kicking accuracy. Hold onto the wall for balance and kick as slowly as possible, concentrating on form. (10 kicks left leg and right leg).

• Front. See Figure 6-34.

• Roundhouse. See Figure 6-35.

• Sidekick. See Figure 6-36.

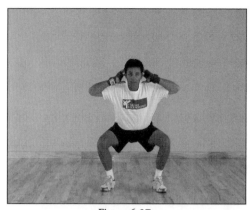

Figure 6-37a

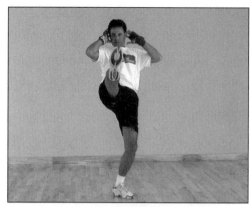

Figure 6-37b

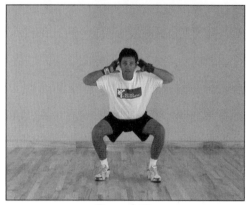

Figure 6-38a

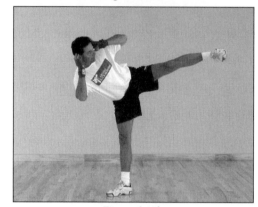

Figure 6-38b

f. Squat/kicks.

- Front. See Figures 6-37a, b.
- Sidekick. See Figures 6-38a, b.

CHAPTER 7

Advanced Techniques

The following techniques are offered for the more advanced or competitive kickboxers. *For your reference, the step number from the original workout described in Chapter 5 is indicated at the beginning of each add-on.*

Step 5. Punches. (refer to page 71)

j. Body punching. The body is a bigger and less mobile target to strike than the head, but getting into position to work on the inside is a typical risk/reward situation. If you take the risk and are able to go to the body with your punches, it takes a toll on your opponent and will eventually wear him out. See Figure 7-1a, b.

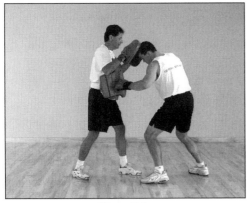

Figure 7-1a

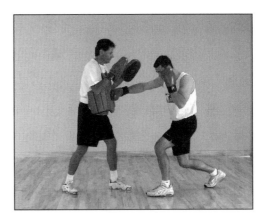

Figure 7-1b

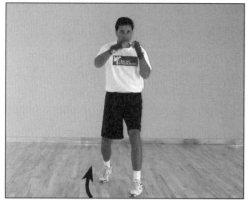

Figure 7-2a

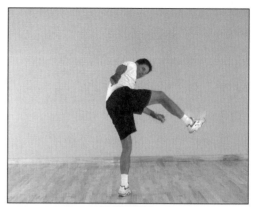

Figure 7-2b

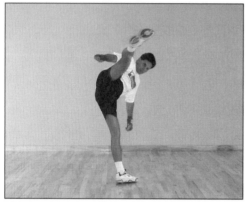

Figure 7-2c

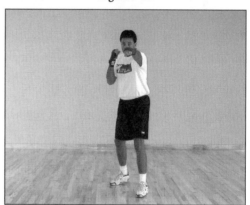

Figure 7-3a

Step 9. Kicks. (refer to page 77)

i. Wheel kick (rear leg). This is a counter kick of secondary importance that is difficult to execute and land and is rarely used in a kickboxing bout since it is not prudent to turn your back on an opponent. However, as with a hook or spinning side, it can surprise an opponent. If it lands, it can be a devastating kick. See Figure 7-2a, b, c.

- Step-through wheel kick (lead leg). Step toward your opponent, spin counter-clockwise and wheel kick with the left leg used offensively.
- Double wheel kick (rear leg, lead leg). Right wheel kick, left wheel kick.

Step 10. Punching and Kicking Combinations. (refer to page 77)

g. Jab/wheel kick, Figures 7-3a, b, c.

h. Jab/cross/step-through wheel kick.

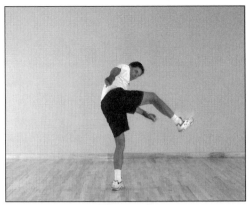

Figure 7-3b

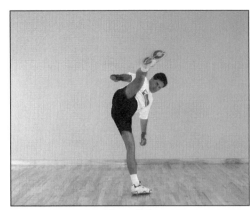

Figure 7-3c

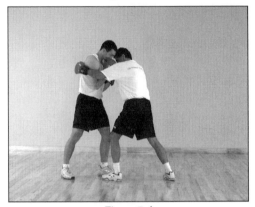

Figure 7-4

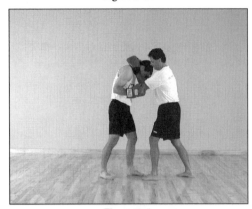

Figure 7-5a

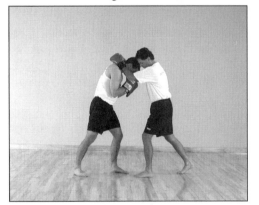

Figure 7-5b

Step 17. Conditioning and Strengthening. (refer to page 84)

    g. Clinching. Hanging on to an opponent is illegal in both boxing and kickboxing, but it is used to rest when tired or to clear your head when hurt. See Figure 7-4.

    h. Neck wrestling. Similar to clinching, but legal in Thai-style boxing to execute knee strikes. See Figures 7-5a, b.

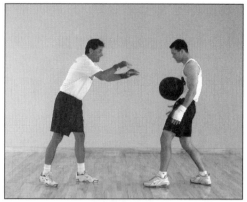

Figure 7-6

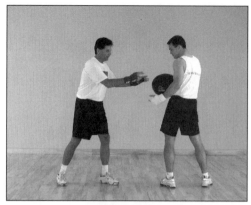

Figure 7-7

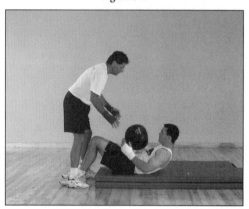

Figure 7-8

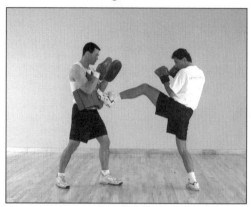

Figure 7-9a

i. Consecutive wheel kicks. Not practical for use in the ring or for self-defense, but good for developing balance.

Other.

a. Medicine ball. Used to strengthen the torso for receiving punches and kicks. Restricted to competitive fighters only. See Figures 7-6, 7-7, and 7-8.

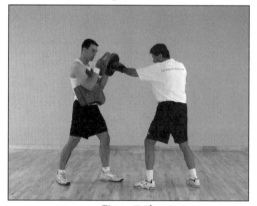

Figure 7-9b

b. Modified sparring. The last step before actual sparring. Puts all the techniques into perspective using a live target. The combinations are limitless, but it's best to practice the basic ones that are the most efficient. See Figures 7-9a, b, c; 7-10a, b, c; and 7-11a, b.

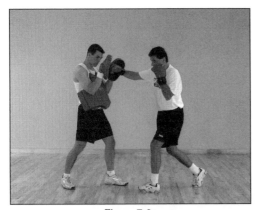

Figure 7-9c

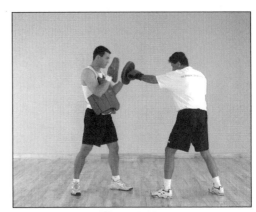

Figure 7-10a

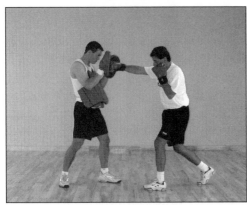

Figure 7-10b

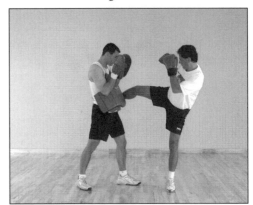

Figure 7-10c

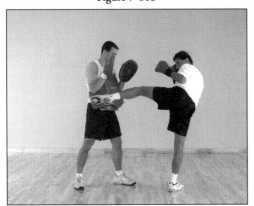

Figure 7-11a

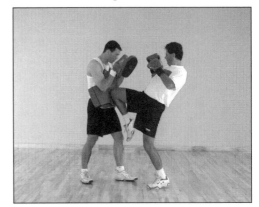

Figure 7-11b

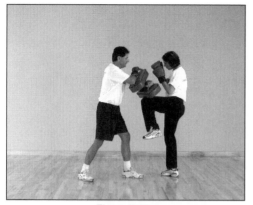

Figure 7-12a

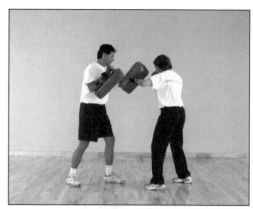

Figure 7-12b

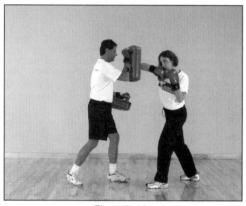

Figure 7-12c

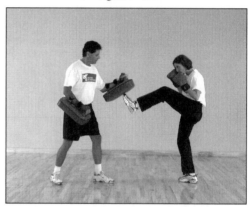

Figure 7-13a

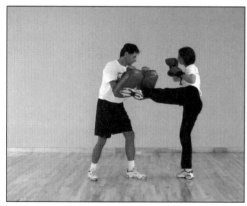

Figure 7-13b

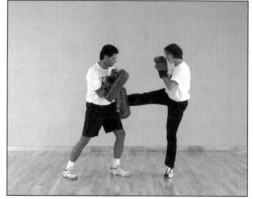

Figure 7-14a

c. Thai pads. Use these to punch *and* kick rather than punch (focus mitts) *or* kick (kicking pad). See Figures 7-12a, b, c; 7-13a, b; and 7-14a, b, c.

• Chest protector and punch mitts.

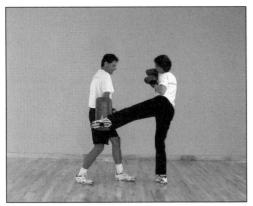

Figure 7-14b

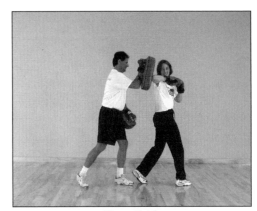

Figure 7-14c

d. Sparring. Sparring is not required as part of the fitness program. Some people, however, want to try sparring to test their skills. This is done outside of the normal class setting and must be supervised by a qualified instructor.

Required Equipment.

- Sparring gloves
- Headgear
- Mouthpiece
- Shin guards
- Foot pads
- Forearm pads
- Groin cup for men or breast protector for women. See Appendix.

CHAPTER 8

Optional Workouts

The following optional workouts can be used to change your basic *Cardio Kickboxing®* routine. The Endurance Workout is particularly useful for beginners since they are required to continually focus on each individual punch and kick through repetition. This helps to quickly improve basic techniques. The Thai-style Workout requires knowledge of the advanced techniques. Additionally, the one-on-one practice with a partner makes the workout more realistic and useful for applying the techniques to an actual person. Finally, the Without Equipment workout format can be used when there is no equipment available due to space or budget limitations. Performing optional workouts, when warranted, helps to keep the *Cardio Kickboxing®* workout fresh, interesting, and motivating especially for experienced participants in the program. Simply stated, the formats are basically the same for each class. The workout phase is where we plug in the optional component as outlined below:

Endurance workout	Thai-Style Workout	Without Equipment Workout
Warm-up	Warm-up	Warm-up
Review	Review	Review
Workout Phase	Workout Phase	Workout Phase
(Repetition of individual punches and kicks on a heavy bag)	*(One-on-one with a partner and with the Thai focus pads)*	*(Extends the review by repetition of patterns while working as a group)*
Conditioning/Strengthening	Conditioning/Strengthening	Conditioning/Strengthening
Tapering/Cool-down	Tapering/Cool-down	Tapering/Cool-down

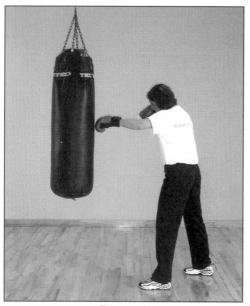

Figure 8-1

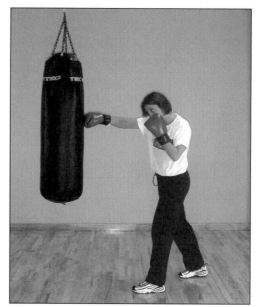

Figure 8-2

A. ENDURANCE WORKOUT

In place of the circuit-training component of the basic format, the endurance workout can be inserted. After the warm-up and review portions (sections 1-11 of the basic workout), each participant uses a heavy bag to work on continuous and repetitive execution of individual techniques. For example, jab 16–24 times consecutively. See Figure 8-1. Then use the right cross punch 16–24 times consecutively. See Figure 8-2. Cover all of the basic punches and kicks. See Figure 8-3 and Figure 8-4. Then move into combinations. This format is a substitute for section 12 of the basic workout (circuit training/bag work) and takes about 20 minutes without a break. It really develops the burn for all major muscle groups. If you have not learned to relax when you execute a punch or a kick, you will quickly fatigue yourself. You must stay loose until the moment of impact and then tighten all your muscles. This approach can also be used to change the normal routine to keep the motivation level high. If there are not enough bags to accommodate all of the participants, they can share a bag while working on the opposite sides. Each partner takes turns holding it for the other. You will then finish your workout by including your normal cool-down procedure. The outline would flow together as follows:

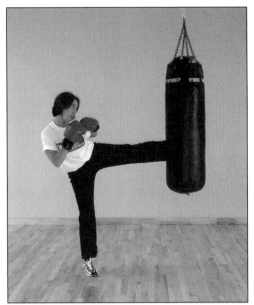

Figure 8-3

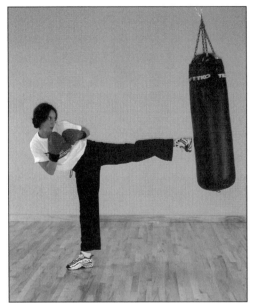

Figure 8-4

Warm-up

Step 1. Warm-up routine

Step 2. Punching drills

Step 3. Stance and foot movement

Step 4. Bobbing and weaving

Review

Step 5. Five basic punches

Step 6. Punching combinations

Step 7. Shadow-boxing

Step 8. Knee-ups

Step 9. Basic kicks

Step 10. Punching and kicking combinations

Workout

Step 11. Shadow kickboxing

Step 12. Endurance Workout (repetition of basics on a heavy bag)

Step 13. Speed punching drills; power punching drills

Step 14. Speed kicking drills; power kicking drills

Step 15. Skipping rope

Step 16. Plyometric exercises

Step 17. Crunches and push-ups

Tapering and Cool-down

Step 18. Upper body stretches

Step 19. Torso and lower body stretches

B. THAI-STYLE WORKOUT

This training format is not suited to beginners since knowledge of the intermediate and advanced techniques is required. A partner of approximately the same height and weight to work with is more suitable. The circuit training on the bags (Step 12 of the basic workout) is substituted with one-on-one drills and Thai focus pads with a partner. The participants are also allowed the option of going barefoot in these types of classes.

A bout for a professional Muay Thai fighter is scheduled for 5 three-minute rounds. Receiving kicks to the legs, elbows to the face, or knee strikes to the body requires incredible amounts of conditioning. We practice these techniques in the advanced *Cardio Kickboxing®* class primarily for self-defense purposes since they are very effective against an attacker. However, safety is a serious consideration. Even though you are not actually sparring, there is the possibility of an accidental injury. Therefore, we recommend the use of protective gear as mentioned at the end of Chapter 7.

It is necessary to first discuss several differences between kickboxing and Muay Thai with regards to the fundamentals at this point.

Stance

A Thai boxer's stance is similar to a kickboxer's stance, but the heel is often raised on the rear foot. See Figure 8-5. Less foot movement is necessary in Thai boxing as compared to that of a kickboxer; a Thai boxer delivers more powerful kicks from a stable stance. A Thai boxer's hands are held a bit higher and more forward than a boxer's hands, which are held by the cheeks. The palms face more toward the opponent, which helps protect against elbow strikes. See Figure 8-6.

Punches

Thai boxers and boxers employ the same basic punches, *i.e.,* jab, cross, hook, and uppercut. Backfists are not normally employed in the sport of Muay Thai or in the Thai-style workout. (Parrying punches and using reinforced palm blocks, is not unusual.) Practicing the use of the various elbows is very common.

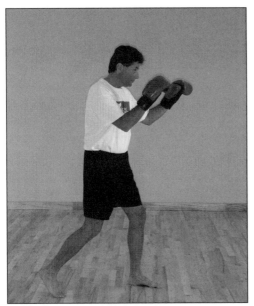

Figure 8-5

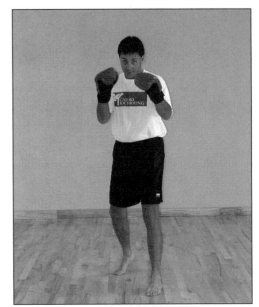

Figure 8-6

Kicks

Switching the lead-leg is more common in Thai boxing than it is in boxing or kickboxing. The front kick, which makes contact with the ball of the foot, is sometimes referred to as a push kick. This kick uses more hip action for penetration. Using the heel of the foot for more thrusting power is also acceptable. The round kick is more of a soccer-style kick that uses the shin as the point of contact rather than the instep. This kick is the primary kick in Thai boxing. There are more target options such as the outside of the leg (quadriceps), inside the leg, calves, and so on. The lead-leg sidekick is occasionally used as a defensive counterkick. Knee strikes are also employed to the body and sometimes to the head by grabbing the opponent's neck. Blocking kicks to the legs using the shin is often practiced as well.

Elbow and Knee Strikes

These techniques are illegal in kickboxing, but they are often practiced in Muay Thai or for self-defense purposes.

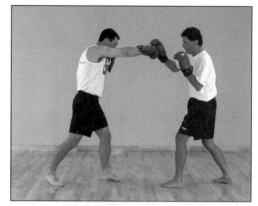

Figure 8-7

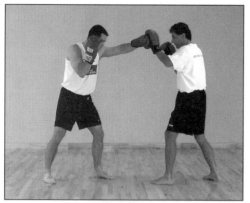

Figure 8-8

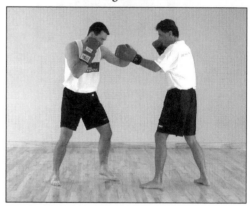

Figure 8-9

Below is a typical Thai-style *Cardio Kickboxing®* workout format:

Warm-up

Step 1. Skipping rope (3 times) two or three minute rounds with a 60-second "rest" period.

Step 2. During the rest period, the participants do a series of ten push-ups, crunches, and squats.

Step 3. Stretching segment.

Review

Step 4. Stance and foot movement.

Step 5. Bobbing and weaving.

Step 6. Basic punches.

Step 7. Elbow strikes.

Step 8. Punching combinations.

Step 9. Shadow-boxing.

Step 10. Shin blocks.

Step 11. Knee strikes.

Step 12. Basic kicks.

Step 13. Shadow kickboxing employing all techniques.

Workout

Step 14. Thai-Style workout (with a partner) Light contact.

Basics (examples)

   a. Punches. Jab (see Figure 8-7), cross punch (see Figure 8-8), hook punch (see Figure 8-9), and uppercut (see Figure 8-10).

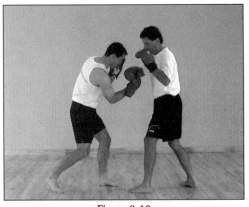

Figure 8-10

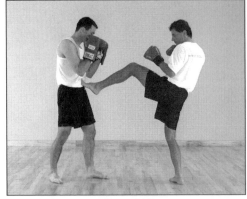

Figure 8-11

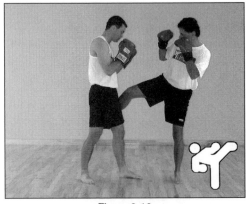

Figure 8-12

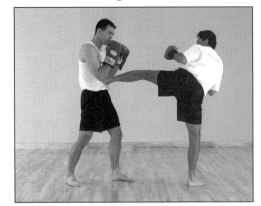

Figure 8-13

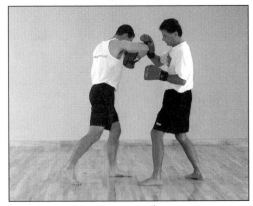

Figure 8-14

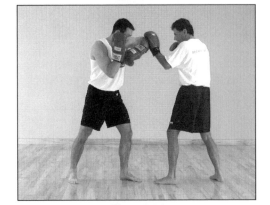

Figure 8-15

b. Kicks. Lead-leg front kick (see Figure 8-11), right round kick (see Figure 8-12) and lead left sidekick (see Figure 8-13).

c. Elbow strikes. Right elbow strike (see Figure 8-14) and left elbow strike (see Figure 8-15).

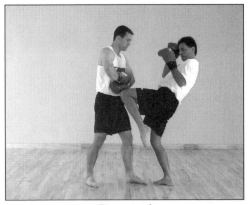

Figure 8-16

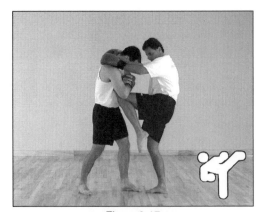

Figure 8-17

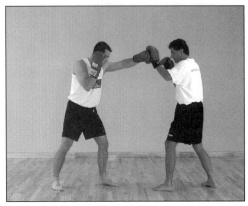

Figure 8-18a

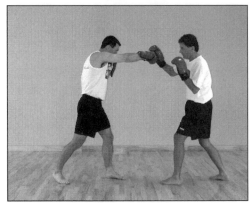

Figure 8-18b

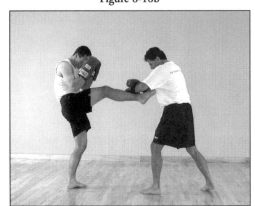

Figure 8-18c

    d. Knee strikes. Outside (see Figure 8-16) and inside (see Figure 8-17).

Punching and kicking combinations (examples)

    a. Left jab (see Figure 8-18a), right cross punch (see Figure 8-18b), and right rear-leg front kick (see Figure 8-18c).

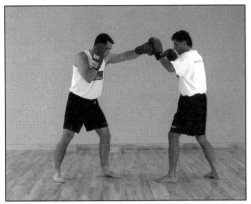

Figure 8-19a

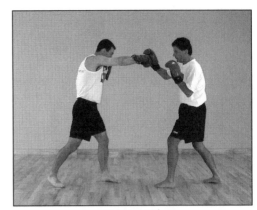

Figure 8-19b

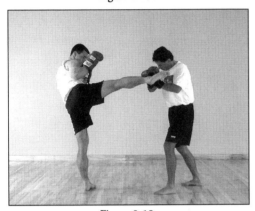

Figure 8-19c

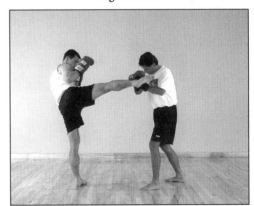

Figure 8-20a

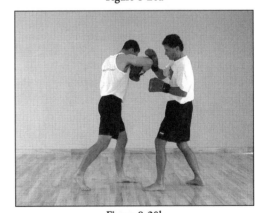

Figure 8-20b

b. Left jab (see Figure 8-19a), right cross punch (see Figure 8-19b), and right round kick (see Figure 8-19c).

c. Right round kick (see Figure 8-20a) and right elbow strike (see Figure 8-20b).

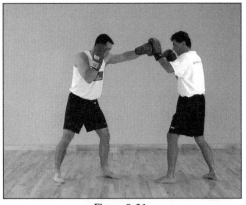

Figure 8-21a

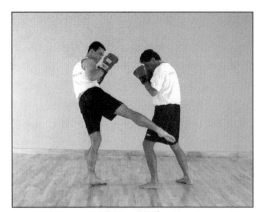

Figure 8-21b

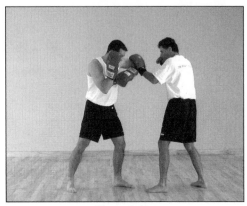

Figure 8-21c

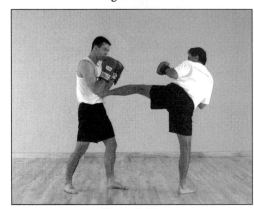

Figure 8-22a

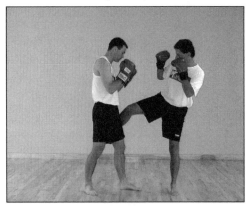

Figure 8-22b

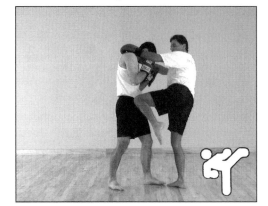

Figure 8-22c

   d. Left jab (see Figure 8-21a), right round kick (see Figure 8-21b), left elbow strike (See Figure 8-21c).

   e. Left side (push) kick (see Figure 8-22a), right round kick (see Figure 8-22b), and neck grab with left knee strike (see Figure 8-22c).

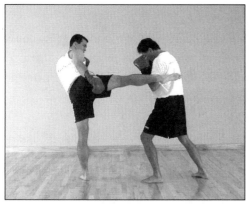

Figure 8-23a

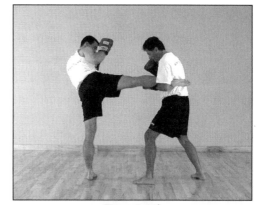

Figure 8-23b

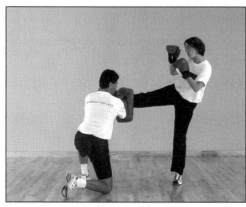

Figure 8-24a

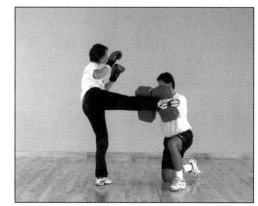

Figure 8-24b

    f. Occasionally practice catching and trapping the leg. (See Figures 8-23a, b).

Step 15. Use of Thai Focus Pads—Use the same or similar combinations. You may also practice low kicks while kneeling. (See Figures 8-24a, 8-24b)

Strengthening and Cool-down

Step 16. Push-ups with a partner applying *light* resistance by pushing on the back of the person doing the push-ups and crunches.

Step 17. Stretching on the mats with a partner applying *light* pressure for more stretch.

C. Workout without Equipment

Another workout format forgoes the use of equipment completely. This strays from the intent of the program since it eliminates the resistance component (bag work) of the original workout. It is useful for learning the basic punches and kicks in the air, but you will need to do a strength training routine using free weights or machines at another time.

Make no mistake about it: these types of workouts are cardiovascularly intense. Since they are set up like aerobics classes that run for 45–60 continuous minutes of non-stop action, there is seldom any time to pause to explain the techniques.

This program is easily be done by extending the warm-up and review portions of the basic workout (sections 1-11 and 13-19), by doing more repetitions, or by adding more conditioning drills or variations as "add-ons" (intermediate and advanced techniques) to the basic workout. This type of workout also tends to be choreographed to the beat of the music. The music should range between 128 and 134 beats per minute. Anything much faster is putting you at risk for injury.

Of course, caution must be used when punching and kicking in the air to avoid hyperextension of the elbows and knees trying to keep up with the speed of movement.

Often, many aerobic instructors teaching this type of class may not have a strong background in kickboxing or the martial arts. They may have a tendency to make up patterns to fill time. This is not necessary since, as mentioned previously, there are many techniques available in the sport to more than provide enough punching and kicking variations during your class.

Half-time vs. Tempo

Most martial arts classes conduct their repetition drills in sets of ten. Aerobics classes use sets of eight. The music in these types of classes is divided into a "32 count phrasing." If you listen carefully to any song, you will be able to distinguish the four-beat sequence. Four beats times eight repetitions equals a 32-beat pattern. Aerobic instructors use this rhythmic count to conduct their classes and do so with the non-equipment version of the *Cardio Kickboxing*® workout as well. Many instructors will also use half-time tempo so that the participants can work on form first (slower execution promotes good form). Then they will pick up the speed by punching and kicking to the actual tempo of the music.

Transitioning

When you complete a sequence of 8, 16, or 24 repetitions or go to another series of combinations, it is necessary to transition from one set to another. You

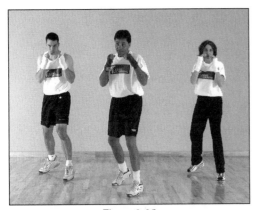

Figure 8-25

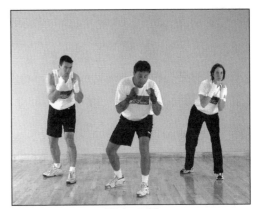

Figure 8-26

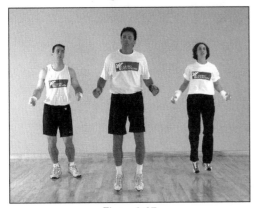

Figure 8-27

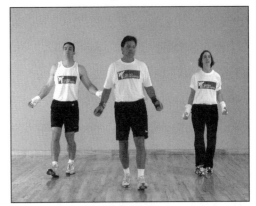

Figure 8-28

can also use transitioning to take a break from a particularly demanding sequence. Some of the transition moves associated with the *Cardio Kickboxing®* workout without Equipment are:

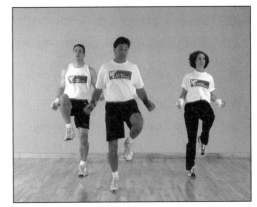

Figure 8-29

- Boxer's shuffle. See Figure 8-25.

- Bobbing and weaving. See Figure 8-26.

- Skipping rope (without the actual rope).

    –Ball of foot. See Figure 8-27.

    –Heel touches. See Figure 8-28.

    –Knees up. See Figure 8-29.

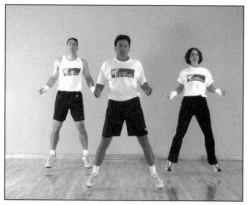

Figure 8-30

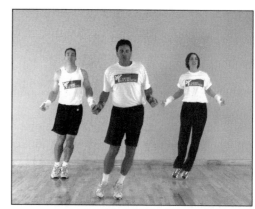

Figure 8-31

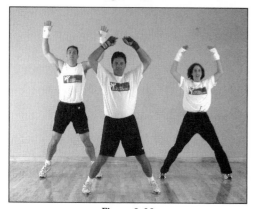

Figure 8-32

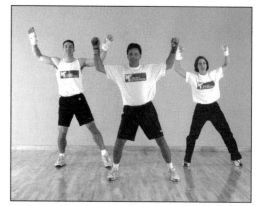

Figure 8-33

–Jacks. See Figure 8-30.

–Ski jump. See Figure 8-31.

- Jumping jacks (see Figure 8-32) or low impact option (see Figure 8-33).

- Shuffle right and left (see Figure 8-34) or shuffle with a sidekick (see Figure 8-35a, b).

- "Flashdance," rapid-fire stepping, and "the moving speed bag" are common transition moves seen in the Tae-Bo videos or other fitness kickboxing-style classes.

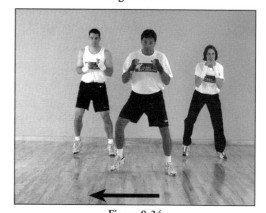

Figure 8-34

Alternating sides

As was previously mentioned, right-handed people who train for boxing and kickboxing rarely switch their lead left leg when training or fighting. In most

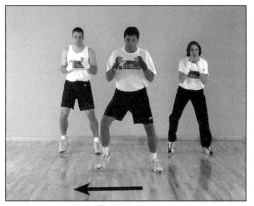

Figure 8-35a

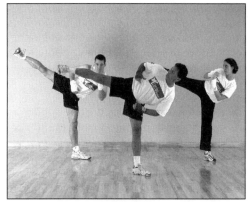

Figure 8-35b

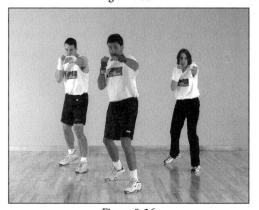

Figure 8-36

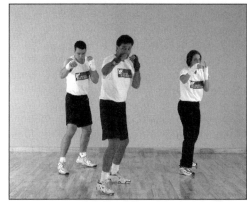

Figure 8-37

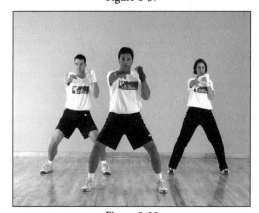

Figure 8-38

group fitness classes, however, the inclination is to work both sides of the body in equal fashion. For example, you will often see participants jabbing with their left hand (see Figure 8-36) and then, for muscle balance, switching their stance to a lead right leg and jabbing with their right hand (see Figure 8-37). You may even see some people punching from what is known in the martial arts as a horse stance, a stance in which both feet parallel to each other. See Figure 8-38. Since the primary goal is for fitness, this is permissible and not unusual.

The following is a sample workout:

Warm-up (Static)

Step 1. Neck.

a. Tilt your head forward and back 4 times; tilt your head left to center and right to center 4 times; turn your head left to center and right to center 4 times, and rotate left to right and right to left 4 times.

Step 2. Upper body.

b. Rotate shoulders forward 4 times and backward 4 times.

c. Stretch up with right arm and pulse 4 times, and repeat with left arm 4 times.

d. Right tricep stretch and left tricep stretch. Hold each for 10 seconds.

e. Right arm stretch horizontally and left arm stretch horizontally. Hold each for 10 seconds.

f. Lock fingers for forward press.

Step 3. Lower body.

g. Squats (8 times).

h. Hamstring stretch and hip flexor push (4 times).

i. Full circular trunk rotation left to right (4 times) and right to left (4 times).

Warm-up, Review, and Workout (Combined)

Step 4. Basic punches.

a. Left jab, 8 times half-time and 8 times tempo.

b. Stepping, left jab and right, 8 times each side, tempo.

c. Right cross, 8 times half-time and 8 times tempo.

d. Left hook, 8 times half-time and 8 times tempo.

e. Double left hook, head/body, 8 times tempo.

f. Right uppercut, 8 times half-time and 8 times tempo.

g. Combine jab/cross punch/hook/uppercut, 8 times half-time and 8 times tempo.

Step 5. Bob and weave.

a. Left, right, down, back, and weave, 4 times left and right.

b. Bob and weave in sequence: left, right, down, back, left and right, 4 times.

Transition to right side lead. Use bob and weave.

Step 6. Basic Punches. Repeat (4a to 4g) right jab, left cross, right hook, left uppercut.

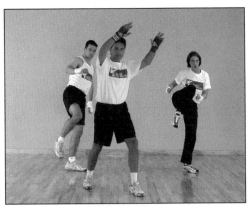

Figure 8-39a

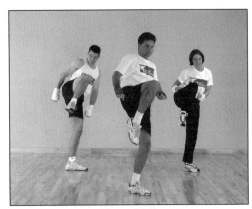

Figure 8-39b

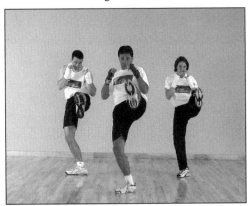

Figure 8-40

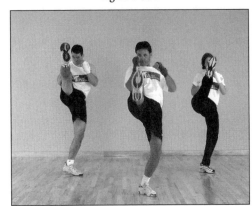

Figure 8-41

a. Moving speed bag, 4 times left and 4 times right.

Step 7. Knee strikes.

a. Left knee strike, 8 times half-time, 16 times tempo, and 8 times half-time.

b. Right knee strike, 8 times half-time, 16 times tempo, and 8 times half-time (see Figures 8-39a, b).

Transition, skipping rope, 4 times each.

Step 8. Front Kicks.

a. Lead-leg left front kick, 8 times half-time, 16 times tempo, and 8 times half-time (see Figure 8-40).

b. Rear-leg right front kick, 8 times half-time, 16 times tempo, and 8 times half-time (see Figure 8-41).

Transition, jumping jacks (16 times).

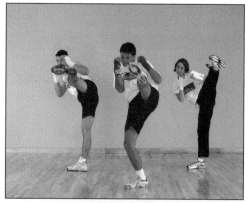

Figure 8-42

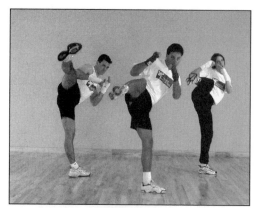

Figure 8-43

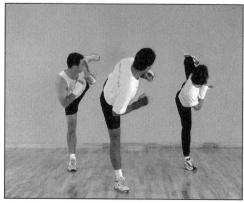

Figure 8-44

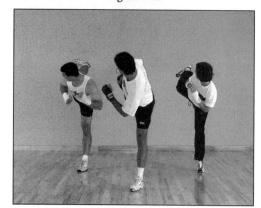

Figure 8-45

Step 9. Roundhouse Kicks.

a. Lead-leg left round kick 8 times half-time, 16 times tempo, and 8 times half-time (see Figure 8-42).

b. Rear-leg right round kick, 8 times half-time, 16 times tempo, and 8 times half-time (see Figure 8-43). Transition, left and right shuffle (4 times).

Step 10. Sidekicks (also referred to as backkicks). Done with a 4 count. Step away (1), step toward the target (2), kick (3), step down (4) (see Figures 8-44 to 8-45).

a. Left leg side, 8 times half-time, 16 times tempo, and 8 times half-time.

b. Right leg sidekick, 8 times half-time, 16 times tempo, and 8 times half-time.

Transition.

a. Left and right shuffle (4 times).

b. Left and right shuffle with sidekick (4 times).

Conditioning and Strengthening

Step 11. Combinations.

a. Left front kick/left jab/right cross/left jab. 4 times half-time, 16 times tempo, and 4 times half-time.

Transition, boxer's shuffle.

b. Right front kick/right jab/left cross/right jab. 4 times half-time, 16 times tempo, and 4 times half-time.

Transition, moving speed bag, 4 times left and 4 times right.

c. Left round kick/left jab/right cross/left jab. 4 times half-time, 16 times tempo, and 4 times half-time.

Transition, boxer's shuffle.

d. Right round kick/right jab/left cross/right jab. 4 times half-time, 16 times tempo, and 4 times half-time.

Transition, flashdance (Use 4 sides of the room: facing front, left, rear, right).

- Legwork only.
- Combine legwork with straight punching and/or uppercuts.

Transition, boxer's shuffle.

e. Double left knee strike/left sidekick/right cross. 4 times half-time, 16 times tempo and 4 times half-time.

Transition, boxer's shuffle.

f. Double right knee strike/right sidekick/left cross. 4 times half-time, 16 times tempo, and 4 times half-time.

Transition, left and right shuffle with sidekick.

g. Left front kick/right back kick. 4 times half-time, 16 times tempo, 4 times half-time.

Transition, boxer's shuffle.

h. Right front kick/left back kick. 4 times half-time, 16 times tempo, and 4 times half-time.

Transition.

a. Skipping rope (4 times each variation).

b. Jumping jacks (16 times).

Note : Conversions may also take place with elbow strikes, knee strikes, back-fists and so on. Plyometrics such as the squat and front kick or lunges can also be added to fatigue the legs even more.

Tapering and Cool-down

The above combinations can be repeated in half-time with less repetitions.

Repeat Steps 1, 2, and 3 above (upper and lower body stretches).

Add crunches and stretching on the mats to finish off the workout.

Should you need to visualize these workout formats, videos are available from a number of sources. Please refer to the Resource Guide on page 149.

Appendix

Basic Equipment List

The following equipment is commonly used to train competitive kickboxers and commonly found in the original *Cardio Kickboxing* ® classes:

EQUIPMENT

- Heavy Bags
- Water-Filled Heavy Bags
- Water-Filled Uppercut Bags
- Free-Standing Heavy Bags
- Speed Bags
- Double-End Bags
- Reflex Bags
- Double-DE Bags
- Thai Heavy Bags (Banana Bags)

Auxiliary Equipment

- Round Timers
- Punch Mitts—regular
    –kickboxing punch mitts
    –Thai pads
- Kickboxing Pads—body shields

Optional Advanced Equipment

- Medicine Balls
- Chest Protectors

Personal Equipment:

- Handwraps
- Bag Gloves
- Jump Ropes
- Head Gear
- Foot Pads
- Shin Pads
- Forearm Pads

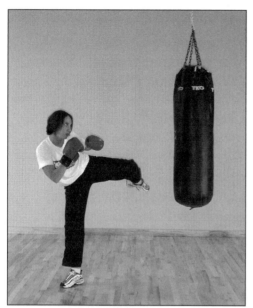

Figure A-1

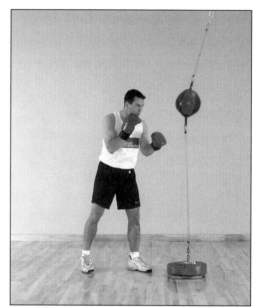

Figure A-2

The amount and type of equipment utilized will vary from individual to individual and from facility to facility. It also depends on what level you want to take the workout. The asterisks above indicate the minimum personal equipment needed for participation in the *Cardio Kickboxing*® fitness program.

To obtain a catalog of this equipment refer to the Resource Guide on page 149.

Equipment Functions

Of Primary Importance:

- **Heavy bag** develops punching & kicking power; improves muscle tone, Figure A-1.
- **Double-end bag** improves punching accuracy, bobbing and weaving, foot movement, Figure A-2.
- **Uppercut bag** improves uppercut; strengthens biceps; can also be used for knee strikes. Figures A-3, A-4.
- **Thai heavy bag** develops kicking power especially for leg kicks, Figure A-5.
- **Jump rope** is used to warm up or for conditioning; great tool for developing coordination.

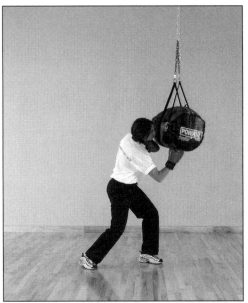

Figure A-3

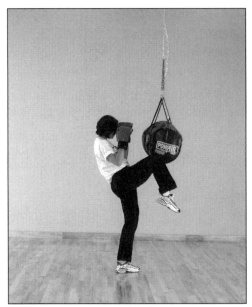

Figure A-4

Of Secondary Importance:

- **Free-standing bag** developed for home use or when unable to hang heavy bags.

- **Speed bag** improves timing, hand speed, hand-eye coordination; strengthens shoulders.

- **Double double-end bag** similar to the regular double-end bag, but provides body and head variations.

- **Chest protector** teaches body punching and permits kicks to the body without injury to the instructor; used in modified sparring to put all the techniques together.

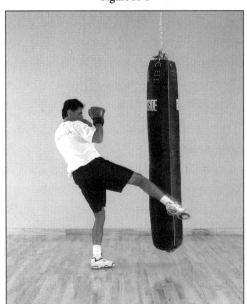

Figure A-5

135

The following tools are used in a *Cardio Kickboxing®* class. If you working at home, it's not likely that you'll be using them unless you have a partner.

- **Punch mitts** develop a sense of distance and angles for a moving target with feedback from the instructor.
- **Kicking pad** develops utilization of kicks for a moving target and sense of distance with feedback from the instructor.
- **Thai pads** develop punching and kicking combinations, use of knees and elbows with feedback from the instructor.

Punch mitts

There are a few methodologies for holding the punch mitts. The one I prefer is the left-to-left; right-to-right method, which encourages the pivoting of the hips and, thus, forces the person punching to use the lower body rather than punch with the shoulders and arms. The punch mitts actually represent two heads instead of one. They should be held in a split fashion at approximately a 45° angle with your elbows bent. When you receive the punch, you must offer an moderate resistance, i.e., not too stiff or too loose. You also have to learn to turn the mitts to accept a hook or uppercut. By holding the punch mitts, you will also develop an ability to read (anticipate) which punch the person is about to throw. Your responsibility is to offer a moving target and give feedback to keep your partner's hands up, check his or her balance, make sure he or she does not cross the feet, and see how he or she reacts when you move forward.

Kicking pad

The kicking pad or air shield is a good tool to learn how to utilize your kicks. You can practice your form in the air and develop power on the heavy bags, but this station is designed to make your kicks effective, not pretty. The person holding the pad has to learn how to rest the pad on the hip. When the pad is directly facing the person kicking, he or she must use a lead or rear leg front kick. The lead-leg sidekick is sometimes used as the person with the pad moves forward. At a side angle, the kicker should use the roundhouse kick. Then the holder offers the pad to mix it up a bit.

Thai pads

The Thai pads and maxi-mitts are the next training step. As a kickboxer, you do not throw single kicks or punches, you kick-and-punch or punch-and-kick. The Thai pads and maxi-mitts are more realistic tools than a heavy bag because you are offering a moving target. You can also introduce knee strikes and elbows to the mix as well. These are heavier than the punch mitts so it is imperative that you are in shape to keep them up. Over time, you may get tendonitis in your shoulders or elbows from holding them. It is an occupational hazard. I have taken over three million punches to these pads in the last eight years and I am still here in one piece.

When taking a beginner on any of the above targets, you should first use the command approach, i.e., you call out the individual punches or kicks. When both you and the person on offense become more comfortable with these training devises, you can use the "you pitch and I will catch method." The person on offense then kicks and punches when he or she sees fit; based on distance and angle of attack, you have to react by catching the kicks and punches on the pads. I think you will be surprised at how much power some lighter weight people can generate who think they do not punch or kick very hard. Conversely, some larger more muscular people push their punches (until they learn the proper technique) and often burn out quickly due to lack of conditioning (until they improve their fitness level). In any event, you should know what you are doing and pay attention. Otherwise, you will get dinged!

The mindset of the person on offense should be that when an attacker crosses the imaginary line and crosses over into his or her personal space, he or she must keep punching and kicking until the person backs off. This attitude can then be transferred to other environments should they become threatened. A person cannot hurt you (unless he or she has a weapon) until your space is invaded. Once that happens, it is all-out war until that person is defeated and the threat is over. You do not get this type of training in an aerobic kickboxing class. It is also legitimate confidence builder rather than false confidence builder because you *know* rather than *feel* your techniques will work.

Overview of International Sport Karate Association Rules and Regulations

For Full-Contact Karate and Kickboxing Competition

1. Full Contact Karate (North American Style Kickboxing)

Full Contact Karate rules permit kicks and punches above the belt only. In addition to approved boxing gloves (8 oz. for 153 lbs. and under, 10 oz. for all weights over 153 lbs.), approved footpads and shin guards are also mandatory. Kicking judges will count kicks for each of the two fighters. Eight kicks are mandatory per round (Minimum Kick Requirement, MKR). A knockdown or standing eight-count is counted as a kick for both fighters.

There is a half-point penalty for each missed kick and disqualification will result for failing to meet the MKR in any two rounds for any match of 6 rounds or less. In bouts that are scheduled for seven to eleven rounds, failing the MKR in any three rounds means disqualification. For a twelve-round bout, if the MKR is not fulfilled in any four rounds, the fighter is disqualified. Sweeps are legal, but must be to the front leg only from the outside in or back to front with the contact being on the foot pad or low calf only. Rounds are two minutes in length with a one-minute rest.

2. Freestyle Rules

Freestyle rules follow the Full Contact Karate format except for the following:

a. Roundhouse-type kicks are allowed to the legs above the knee.

b. There is no minimum kick requirement.

c. Foot pads and shin guards are optional for professional fighters.

d. If one fighter elects to wear footpads, his opponent must also wear them.

e. Thai-style shorts are encouraged in these bouts.

f. Sweeps are allowed to the inside or outside of the front or back leg.

3. Oriental Rules

Oriental rules follow the freestyle rules except for the following:

a. Roundhouse kicks are allowed to any part of the leg except for the knee.

b. Foot pads and shin guards are not allowed to be used.

c. Shorts are mandatory.

d. Knee strikes are permitted to the body.

e. Limited neck wrestling is allowed.

f. Rounds are usually three minutes in length.

g. World title fights are usually eight rounds.

4. Thai-Style Rules (Muay Thai)

Thai rules follow the Oriental rules except for the following:

    a. Knees may be permitted to the leg.

    b. Elbow strikes, with the exception of the spinning elbow, may be permitted.

    c. Hook kicks and spinning hook kicks may be used to the legal targets on the legs.

    d. All title fights will be five rounds in length.

    e. A two-minute rest period between rounds may be permitted.

5. Chinese Style Rules (San Shou)

Chinese style rules follow freestyle rules with an emphasis on throws and takedowns for extra points.

Amateur Matches

Amateur matches will usually be sanctioned under Full-Contact Karate and freestyle rules only. All amateur fighters are required to wear approved headgear, footpads, and shin guards in addition to standard equipment. Pre-made hand-wraps (without tape) approved by the ISKA representative may be allowed. All other rules apply as per professional Full-Contact Karate and freestyle matches. Most amateur matches consist of three two-minute rounds, with one-minute rest periods. With the approval of the ISKA, amateur title matches may be four or five rounds in duration. Novice fighters may be permitted to fight rounds of one and a half minutes per round, with the approval of the ISKA representative. Under no circumstances may amateur fighters receive a purse.

To purchase the *ISKA Official Rules And Regulations Handbook*, please call: 1-352-375-8144.

Glossary of Kickboxing Terms

Athletic Performance

The five components needed to improve athletic performance are: skill, speed, stamina, strength, and psyche. Improving athletic performance is often confused with improving physical fitness by the general public.

Backfist (punch)

For right-handed people, it is thrown with the back of the right hand after spinning clockwise on the left foot. Elbow is kept bent. Also can be thrown stepping through and spinning counter-clockwise using the left hand. A double-spinning backfist is thrown with the right first, then left.

Blocks

Conventional martial arts blocks are not used in kickboxing. The most effective defensive maneuvers are foot movement, bobbing and weaving, and keeping your hands up. See also forearm blocks, foot movement, parrying, and shin blocks, below.

Bobbing and Weaving

Head movements used to avoid a slip punch. Movements are taught in sequence to help memorize the six basic options. Left (45°), right (45°), straight down, lean back, weave left, weave right. Used more frequently in boxing than kickboxing.

Body Punching

Attacking the body with punches. Wears down an opponent whose torso area has not been strengthened with crunches, the medicine ball, or Nautilus machines. Bigger target area than the head, but difficult to get "inside" to hit.

Cardio Kickboxing®

A fitness program created by Frank Thiboutot that is also a registered trademark owned by Sport Karate, Inc. The program is based on authentic *sport-specific* kickboxing techniques which are somewhat modified to suit the general 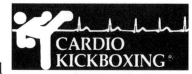 public interested in this type of workout for its fitness and self-defense benefits. The original program (1992) is equipment intensive. The modified program (1999) is an optional format without equipment that can be used as an introductory workout.

Circuit Training (Bag Work)

Stations of various pieces of equipment used in boxing and kickboxing gyms that develop both skill and power. This format increases cardiovascular endurance and provides resistance training. Participants workout using a timer set for 2 or 3 minute rounds with a 15, 30, 45, or 60 second rest period to replicate a kickboxing bout.

Clinching

Holding on or grabbing the arms to prevent an opponent from punching. Illegal in the sports of boxing and kickboxing.

Combinations

There are numerous punching sequences or combinations, kicking combinations, and punching and kicking combinations used in training. However, in kickboxing bouts, the basic and direct combinations as detailed in Chapter 5 are primarily used.

Cool Down

A series of safe stretches particularly, for the lower back area, at the end of every class to begin cooling down. Ex., while lying on the floor with knees bent and both palms on the floor, slowly drop the legs to the left, look right and then reverse the order. Stretching helps to reduce muscle soreness and maintain flexibility.

Cross (punch)

For right-handed people, the power punch thrown with leverage from the torque of the hip and push with the right leg. Hand is palm down when extended with the opposite hand kept at the temple when not being thrown. *Caution, do not hyperextend.* Thrown primarily toward the opponent's chin. Can also be thrown to the body.

Cross Training Shoes

Best suited athletic footwear for aerobic kickboxing classes. Running shoes have too much tread for turning or skipping rope.

Crunches

Used to strengthen the abdominal area. Must be performed slowly and safely. Keep tension on the abs throughout each set without allowing the shoulders to touch the floor.

Caution: Do not pull the neck forward with the hands when fatigued.

Cutting Off (the ring)

To try to prevent an opponent from "running", anticipate the direction that he is about to circle and step into that line. Be prepared to punch at that moment.

Elbow Strikes

Offensive strikes using the elbow which are illegal under Full Contact (American style kickboxing) rules, but are legal in Muay Thai (Thai boxing) rules. The basic elbow strikes are shown in the "Intermediate Techniques" section of this book.

Feinting

Faking or drawing an opponent into reacting to catch him off guard.

Fitness

The five components of physical fitness are cardiorespiratory fitness, muscular strength, muscular endurance, body composition, and flexibility.

Foot Movement

Increases cardiovascular conditioning and ability to move out of harm's way.

- Bouncing: on the balls of the feet without jumping used to warm up the calves.
- Circling: move left or right keeping the lead leg forward.
- Lateral movement: stepping left or right at an angle.
- Pivoting: use the forward foot to pivot either left or right.
- Sliding: always keep the lead foot ahead of the rear foot; avoid crossing the feet.

Forearm Blocking

Hands are held at cheek height with forearms held close to the body to protect the ribs from a kick or punch. Used by kickboxers instead of traditional blocks to defend against body punching and kicks to the torso.

Front Kick

The knee must first be raised and the foot is extended straight out using the ball of the foot with toes curled back as the contact point. Can be used as a "jab" with the left foot for speed and as a "cross" with the right foot for power, for right-handed people.

Group Fitness Classes

Group fitness classes (often referred to as aerobic classes) are most often one hour in duration. Although the content of the class may vary, they should all contain the following components: Warm-Up, Review and Workout Phase, Conditioning and Strengthening Phase, Tapering Phase and Cool-Down.

Handwrapping

The placement of a specially designed cloth (or gauze with tape) on the hands to cover the knuckles, reinforce the wrists, and help to protect the hands from injury. Worn in conjunction with bag gloves.

Hook Kick

A minor kick used with the lead leg. Elevate the leg diagonally toward the right, for right-handed people, at a 45° angle. Retract the foot using the heel or bottom of the foot as the contact point. Caution: could pull the hamstring if target is stable. Only occasionally used in the sport of kickboxing.

Hook (punch)

For right-handed people, the lead hook is thrown with the left hand. It is necessary to pivot on the left foot to synchronize the lower body with the punch for more power.

Can be thrown palm down (using more shoulder and lats) or palm facing (using more bicep). Forearm should not rise above parallel. Can also be thrown with right hand. Thrown in a tight semi-circle with a compact motion to the head or body.

Inside/Outside

As in *inside* techniques vs. *outside* techniques: In reference to an opponent (or an attacker), inside means in close proximity where outside means at a distance. For examples, hooks and uppercuts are usually thrown on the inside; jabs and crosses are usually thrown from the outside. Knee strikes are usually thrown on the inside; kicks are usually thrown from the outside.

Jab (punch)

For right-handed people, the lead punch with the left hand. Executed with speed palm down. Must step with the left foot 4" to 6" toward the target and "snap" the punch for more power. Caution: Do not hyperextend. Used to gauge distance and "set-up" an opponent for other more powerful attacks. Retracts to the side of the face to protect the head when not being thrown. Primarily thrown toward the opponent's chin or nose.

Kickboxing

A sport coming under the umbrella of martial arts whereby fighters are matched according to their weight and experience levels. The rules are similar to a boxing match with kicking allowed as a legal offensive technique. There are five basic systems of rules and regulations for professionals and modifications for amateurs. See Appendix for more details.

Kicking Pad

Used in this program for learning how to *utilize* the kicks rather than for power.

Knee Strikes

Knee strikes are illegal in Full-Contact Karate (American style kickboxing), but legal in Thai-style bouts. They can be thrown from the *outside*, but are more commonly thrown from the *inside* while "neck wrestling" (grabbing the opponent's neck). Very effective for self-defense.

Knee-Ups

Done by bringing the knee up and into the chest to stretch the hamstrings and glutes. Also, used to train for the first step in initiating kicks. Front, inside-out, outside-in, combined inside-out; outside-in.

Leg Checking

Using the bottom of the foot to prevent a person from throwing a kick, particularly a front kick. Okay to use for self-defense; illegal in a sanctioned kickboxing bout.

Maxi-Mitts

Large hand held target pads to offer moving targets for both punching and kicking. Helps to gauge distance and practice hitting a moving target with basic combinations.

Medicine Ball

Used to strengthen the abdominal and torso areas of fighters. Nautilus machines are preferred unless a person intends to compete in boxing or kickboxing.

Modified Sparring

Instructor uses punch mitts and puts on protective gear such as headgear, mouthpiece, chest protector, forearm guards, shin pads, etc. to allow the student an opportunity for a more realistic workout without getting hurt. Not necessary for the scope of fitness kickboxing classes. Used mostly for private students and would-be fighters.

Parrying

Used to deflect a jab. Done with a partially open rear hand (right), not a push.

Plyometric Exercises

Strength movements used to develop powerful quadricep muscles for more explosive kicks.

Punch Mitts

Hand-held target pads used by an instructor to offer moving targets with feedback from an instructor to correct technique. Mitts are separated to encourage "twisting" and use of the hips and legs to develop stronger punches. Helps gauge distance and provide more realism than a punching bag.

Punching and Weaving

Used to avoid "posing" (or freezing to admire one's work) after throwing a punching combination. After finishing a sequence with the right hand, weave to the left. After finishing a sequence with the left hand, weave to the right.

Roundhouse Kick

The knee has to be raised as you pivot on the supporting foot to rotate the hips. The toes are "pointed" and the top of the shoe (laces) are the contact point. Can be thrown with either leg. Similar to the upper body hook (punch) with the left as a lead kick and the right being more powerful. The primary target is the opponent's hip area in Full-Contact Karate (American-style kickboxing) and the quads in Muay Thai.

Shadow Boxing/Kickboxing

Combines hand and/or hand-foot combinations to simulate sparring. Good for conditioning and training to make movement and combinations more fluid and polished.

Shin Blocking

Using the shin to block kicks thrown to the legs. Employed by Thai-style fighters or for self-defense.

Shin Kicks

The roundkick, used by Thai-style fighters, that strikes with the shin instead of the instep. It is best described as more of a "soccer-style" kick for power rather than a hinging-retracted roundhouse kick used by most martial artists.

Side Kick—Lead Leg

For right-handed people, it is thrown with the lead leg (left). The knee must initially be retracted toward the chest. When extended, the heel is the primary point of contact. The leg is again retracted to the chest before being re-placed on the floor. A momentary lateral shift is necessary to utilize the hips to execute this kick. Used to "set up" the hands or as a "stopper" to prevent a rushing type of attack. The midsection is the primary target.

Side Kick—Spinning

Same basis criteria as the front leg side kick. For right handed people, it is thrown with the right leg after spinning clockwise on the left supporting foot and picking up your target over the right shoulder. The midsection is the primary target area.

Skipping Rope

Great conditioning and coordination tool. Done primarily with only a slight bend of the knees without leaving the floor more than an inch unless doing tricks or power jumps (not the same as the conventional schoolyard jump).

Slow Motion Kicking

Used to specifically stress muscles for each basic kick. Increases accuracy and improves kicking form.

Stance

Natural boxers/kickboxers stance, not the deep static stances found in traditional martial arts classes. Both feet are approximately hip distance apart; not too narrow, wide, or deep, which hampers mobility or stability. For right-handed people, the left foot is nearly straight ahead; the right foot is at a 45° angle. The chest is at an angle between 30° and 45°.

Stretch Kicking

Straight-leg stretch kicks that can be used to further stretch the legs after first using the knee ups. Front, inward, outward, and lateral motions. For safety reasons, the should never be used for beginners.

Thai Pads

Focus pads used to practice punching, kicking, elbow, and knee strikes.

Training Gloves

Also referred to as bag gloves. Similar to boxing gloves in shape, but uses Velcro to secure the gloves instead of laces. 12 oz. to16 oz. and durable. Used to protect the hands from injury when striking punching bags or punch mitts. Not to be used for sparring.

Training Guidelines

To improve anyone's level of fitness, the following five criteria must be considered in setting up any training schedule or program: frequency, intensity, duration, mode of activity, and resistance training.

Uppercut (punch)

Necessary to bend at the knees for leverage and more power. Thrown palm facing the body with either hand as perpendicular as possible to the floor. Thrown in a tight compact fashion. Target is the chin or solar plexus.

Warm-up

Non-ballistic movements used to warm the muscles before engaging in more strenuous physical activity.

Wheel Kick

A minor, albeit, powerful kick with the rear leg. For right-handed people, spin clockwise on the left supporting foot, elevate the straight right leg as you locate the target over the right shoulder. Strike with the heel or the bottom of the foot. (Practicing this kick on a heavy bag is not recommended; it may stress the hamstring or knee). Also can be done with a bent leg or the side of the foot as the point of contact. Virtually never used in a kickboxing bout, however.

Exercise and Fitness Associations

- ACSM—American College of Sports Medicine
  P.O. Box 1440
  Indianapolis, IN 46206-1440
  (317) 637-9200

- AFPA—American Fitness Professionals & Associates
  P.O. Box 214
  Ship Bottom, NJ 08008
  (609) 978-7583

- IFKA—International Fitness Kickboxing Association
  100 NW 82nd Avenue, Suite 204
  Plantation, FL 33324
  (954) 472-0630

- ISKA—International Sport Karate Association
  P.O. Box 90147
  Gainesville, FL 32607
  (352) 374-6876

- Institute for Aerobic Research
  12330 Preston Road
  Dallas, TX 75230
  (214) 701-8001

- NASPE—National Association for Sport & Physical Education
  1501 16th Street N.W.
  Washington, DC 20036
  (202) 797-4330

- National Strength and Conditioning Association
  P.O. Box 38909
  Colorado Springs, CO 80937
  (719) 632-6722

Sanctioning Bodies for the Sport of Kickboxing

- **ISKA** (International Sport Kickboxing Association), www.iska.com

- **IKF** (International Kickboxing Federation), www.ikfkickboxing.com

- **WKA** (World Karate Association), www.worldkickboxing.com

- **USKBA** (U. S. Kick Boxing Association), www.uskba.com

Resource Guide

Audio Tapes and CDs

- Sports Music
  Box 769689
  Roswell, GA 30076
  (800) 878-4764

- Dynamix
  733 W. 40th St., #10
  Baltimore, MD 21211
  (800) 843-6499

- Power Music
  500 W. 220 South, #200
  Salt Lake City, UT 84101
  (800) 777-2328

Fitness Kickboxing Videos

- *Cardio Kickboxing*® Videos
  Sport Karate, Inc.
  17 Foreside Road
  Cumberland Foreside,
  ME 04110
  (207) 781-2560

Fitness Videos

- Collage Video
  5390 Main Street N.E.
  Minneapolis, MN 55421
  (800) 433-6769

Martial Arts Videos

- Panther Productions
  1010 Calle Negocio
  San Clemente, CA 92673
  (800) 332-4442

Equipment and Product Catalogs

- Century Martial Art Supply
  1705 National Blvd.
  Midwest City, OK 73110
  (800) 626-2787

- Ringside Products, Inc.
  Box 14171
  Lenexa, KS 66285-4171
  (877) 426-9464

- Technical Knockout, Inc.
  P.O. Box 0035 Ellicot Sta.
  Buffalo, NY 14205
  (800) 267-4886

Martial Arts Magazines

- Rainbow Publications
  (Black Belt, Karate/Kung Fu Illustrated, Martial Arts Training)
  24715 Avenue Rockefeller, P.O. Box 918
  Santa Clarita, CA 91380-9018
  (805) 257-4066

Nutrition and Fitness Information

- Covert Bailey Fitness books and videos:
  http://www.healthcentral.com/fitorfat/fitorfat.cfm

Instructor Certification

For *Cardio Kickboxing*® instructor certification, contact:
- Marcus DeValentino, Program Director
  98-1746-B Ka'ahumanu Street
  Pearl Street, HI 96782
  (808) 455-2253
  http://home.hawaii.rr.com/dssi
  devalentino@hawaii.rr.com

Bibliography

ACSM's Position Stand on the Recommended Quantity and Quality of Exercise for Developing and Maintaining Cardiorespiratory and Muscular Fitness in Healthy Adults, MSSE 30:6, William & Wilkins, Baltimore, MD., 1998.

Cooper, Kenneth H. *The Aerobics Way,* Bantam Books, 1977.

ISKA Official Rules and Regulations Handbook, International Sport Karate Association, Gainesville, FL., 1994.

Judy Klemesrud. "Karate's Unlikely First Family," *New York Times,* October 13,1982. as quoted in "Muay Thai Kickboxing History," http://www.theoctagon.com, April 12, 2000.

Lee, Linda. *Bruce Lee: The Only Man I Knew,* Berkeley, CA, 1996. Quoted in Jeff Chen, http://www.ocf.berkeley.edu/~chenj/brucelee/brucelee.html, March 5, 2000).

Makenna Delaney & Sullivan, Inc., Carlsbad, CA., 1996.

Parker, Leilani. *Ed Parker's Kenpo Karate,* 1998. As quoted in www.edparkerikka.com, March 2, 2000.

Report of the Surgeon General, Physical Activity and Health, U.S. Dept. of Health and Human Services, Center for Disease Control, 1996.

Scharff Olson, Michele, Ph.D., FACSM and Henry Williford, Ed.D., FACSM, "Martial Arts Exercise," *ACSM's Health and Fitness Journal,* December 1999.

Seabourne, Tom. Ph.D., *Complete CardioKickboxing,* YMAA Publication Center, 1999.

Thiboutot, Frank. "U.S. Kickboxing Team Competes in Mainland China," *World Competitor Magazine,* October, 1998.

Yang, Jwing-Ming. *Shaolin White Crane,* YMAA Publication Center, 1996.

Zubukovee, R. and P.M. Tiidus. "Physiological and Anthropometric Profile of Elite Kickboxers," *Journal of Strength and Conditioning Research* 9(4): 240–242, 1998.

About The Author

Frank Thiboutot's experiences span three decades with involvement in every aspect of the martial arts. He began boxing in high school in 1966 and began training in the martial arts in 1969. Frank taught karate at the University of Southern Maine in 1970 and at the University of Kabul in Afghanistan in 1973 as a Peace Corps Volunteer. Later, from 1974–1976, Frank studied Tae Kwon Do while serving another two years in the Peace Corps in South Korea.

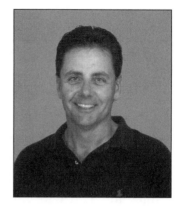

Frank received his 2nd degree black belt in Shoto Kan Karate in September 1975 and his 4th degree black belt in Tae Kwon Do in April 1978.

Frank became involved in Full Contact Karate (American style kickboxing) in 1979 as a trainer, cornerman, and manager of amateur and professional kickboxers. In fact, he managed the entire career of three-time world champion, Danny Melendez. He is a certified "A" rated judge by the International Sport Karate Association (ISKA).

Following are additional highpoints in Frank's career.

- Incorporated Sport Karate, Inc. May, 1984.
- Initiated a bill which became law for the State of Maine to regulate kickboxing by the Maine Athletic Commission, July 1986.
- Appointed ISKA northeast regional representative, June 1990.
- Began promoting professional kickboxing events, 1985.
- Promoted eight title fights televised by FNN/Score, ESPN, and SportsChannel America.
- Hired to give color commentary for several televised shows.
- Matchmade world title fights between U.S. and European fighters.
- Traveled extensively to Canada, the Far East, Europe, the former Soviet Union, and the Caribbean in various capacities relative to the professional side of the sport.
- Opened the first *Cardio Kickboxing*® studio in the Bay Club, One City Center, Portland, Maine to offer "fitness kickboxing" workouts to the general public, October, 1992.

The *Cardio Kickboxing*® logo was first used and the *Cardio Kickboxing*® video was produced for retail distribution, 1993.

- Moved to a larger location at Lifestyle Fitness Center in Portland and began developing the *Cardio Kickboxing®* Certification Program, 1996.

- Began the process of sourcing private label products. Also, in the planning stages are turn-key *Cardio Kickboxing®* studio franchises which will be offered for sale to the general public as will the **Gym-in-the-Box**, a home version of the *Cardio Kickboxing®* workout program, 1997.

Other Awards and Accomplishments:

Invited by the Shanxi Tackunobo Association to organize a first-ever five-man U.S. Team of San Shou style fighters to compete against teams from China and Japan in Taiyuan City, Shanxi Province, People's Republic of China, February, 1998.

- Named the Kickboxing Instructor of the Year for 1997 and inducted into the WKU (World Karate Union) Hall of Fame. June, 1998.

- Produced the *TKO Boxing Workout* video for the TKO Sports Group, July 1998.

- Instructor certification program included in Ringside and Century Martial Arts catalogs, September 1999.

- Provided value-added coupons for K-Tel's *Kickboxing Mix* CD with 50,000 units distributed in retail outlets such as Best Buy, K-Mart, Musicland, etc., October 1999.

About the Models

Lisa D. Lewis, after receiving her B.A. in Communications and English from the University of Southern Maine, was ISKA and APFA certified to teach *Cardio Kickboxing®* in December of 1997. She has enjoyed sharing the sport within a fitness setting ever since.

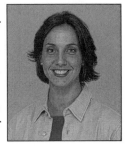

Lisa is currently teaching at three fitness facilities in the Portland, ME area. The classes include a diverse group of individuals that range from energetic teens to dedicated seniors. According to Lisa, "In utilizing bags, gloves, punching mitts, and kicking pads within the classes, we exercise proper technique while continually challenging ourselves in order to foster a fun and safe environment. I've found that for myself and for many others, *Cardio Kickboxing®* is by far the most fun that one can have while participating in a safe and effective workout."

David Lawhorn has enjoyed a notable career as both a kickboxer and boxer. As an amateur kickboxer, he was undefeated; as a boxer, his record was 60–8 (35 by knockout). He was named Maine's "Fighter of the Year" three years in a row. Highlights of David's career include:

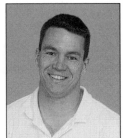

1995 • Vermont Golden Gloves Champion
- New England Golden Gloves Champion (Outstanding Boxer Award)
- New England ABF Champion
- U.S. Region 1 Champion (includes New England, New York, New Jersey)
- Bronze Medal National Golden Gloves Champion (Sportsmanship Award)

1996 • New England Golden Gloves Champion
- Member of U.S. National Team vs. Korea
- Ranked #2 in U.S. by USABF
- ISKA North American Champion

1998 • David turned Professional
- WWKA Undefeated World Champion
- Ranked #1 in World by PKF
- Ranked #2 in World by ISKA
- Ranked #4 in World by IKF

1999 • Retired

SAMPLE TRAINING SCHEDULE IN A STUDIO OR AT HOME

Date										
Shadow Boxing										
Shadow Kickboxing										
Speed Bag										
Heavy Bag										
Reflex Bag										
Double-End Bag										
Thai Heavy Bag										
Dbl. Double-End Bag										
Uppercut Bag										
Punch Mitts/Thai Pads										
Kicking Pad										
Skipping Rope										
Daily Total:										

Index

BOOKS & VIDEOS FROM YMAA

YMAA Publication Center Books

YMAA Publication Center Videotapes

YMAA PUBLICATION CENTER 楊氏東方文化出版中心

4354 Washington Street Roslindale, MA 02131

1-800-669-8892 • ymaa@aol.com • www.ymaa.com